The Meta- bolic Storm

The science of your
metabolism
and why it's
making you fat

P.S. It's not your fault

Emily Cooper, M.D.

Published 2013
ISBN: 978-0-9896902-0-1
Library of Congress Control Number: 2013913572

For information, address:
Seattle Performance Medicine
400 N. 34th St., Suite 300
Seattle, WA 98103

To my grandmother, Ella K. Cooper, M.D.

Contents

Introduction

THIS IS NOT A DIET BOOK.

I won't tell you that eating less, exercising more, juicing kale, or tracking "calories in, calories out" with the latest apps will solve a weight problem.

Why not?

Because of the thousands of patients I've treated over the past twenty-five years, only an alarming few have experienced long-term resolution of their weight problems as a result of dieting and exercising.

But don't worry—there's good news! In the pages to follow, I will share with you what I have learned in my many years of medical practice regarding weight and metabolism. Great scientific advances have been made in recent years that have helped to explain how hormones and metabolism regulate weight gain and loss. For the treatment of obesity, today's science brings great hope.

BECOMING SHERLOCK HOLMES

I'm a Seattle-based physician, board certified in three specialties: Family Medicine, Sports Medicine, and Obesity Medicine. As a medical student training in London, I was exposed to a *systems* approach to medicine, where diagnosis and treatment focus on the body as a whole rather than a fragmented system made up of individual parts. For example, I learned to examine a patient's abdomen as part of the *entire* gastrointestinal system, including the eyes, mouth, hands, and neck. In contrast, when U.S. medical students are asked to examine a patient's abdomen, their exam starts and ends with the abdomen.

While in London, I also learned to diagnose conditions by talking with patients and taking careful patient histories—not just identifying physical signs of disease, but exploring the underlying causes of disease. This approach takes time, patience, and the curiosity to explore the grey areas that exist between health and disease. It is like detective work. In the U.S., I've found that this kind of in-depth exploration is difficult to perform; our average seven-minute doctor-patient interaction leaves little time for deeper investigative work and exploration of those grey areas.

I began to learn about weight and metabolic issues in the 1980s, during my family medicine residency program. This was a period during which preventive medicine was the newest movement in medical care. Researchers were discovering that several health conditions were associated with increased body weight. They had just learned that type 2 diabetes was actually preventable, and that it was associated with insulin resistance and metabolic syndrome. Ultimately, researchers linked the causes of diabetes, cholesterol problems, high blood pressure, and overweight conditions together as one larger condition. They referred to it as "syndrome X" at the time; later, they began to call it "metabolic syndrome" or "dysmetabolic syndrome."

I was very excited to learn about insulin resistance and metabolic syndrome, because if they were indeed reversible and preventable, we had found a new avenue for making a real difference in preventing weight problems, diabetes, heart attacks, and strokes. My interest in this area of medicine grew in the 1990s, when some of my patients were gaining weight even though they were trying to lose or maintain weight. Some of them appeared to be affected by all of the conditions that make up metabolic syndrome; some were affected by only a few of them. Other patients were very healthy, yet they still had problems controlling their weight. Many of my patients kept highly detailed records about what they ate, their exercise regimen, how much they slept, and so on—and in the majority of cases, this meticulously collected data didn't add up based on the conventional "calories in, calories out" theory. This caught my attention, and it became a puzzle that I am still investigating to this day.

DEAD ENDS

Twenty years ago, I thought that all I needed to do to help my overweight patients lose weight was educate them on healthy eating and exercise. This was naïve of me. Granted, at the time (like in the present), this was the standard approach—but it was a short-term strategy at best. Some patients experienced no change in weight whatsoever; others experienced drastic drops in weight of up to one hundred pounds. Regardless of how much weight was lost, however, it always came back. The more patients I treated, the clearer it became: this approach was not working. I was frustrated. It was discouraging to both my patients and me to find that even if we succeeded in the short term, the weight that was lost—and often even more than that—eventually returned.

USING AN OLYMPIC MINDSET

When the diet and exercise approach failed me, I decided to put my sports science experience to use. Sports science focuses on finding out what makes athletes tick in order to help them reach goals like a personal best, breaking a world record, getting to the Olympics, winning a medal, or making a professional team. With this focus in mind, in 1999 I launched a more scientific approach to tackle my patients' weight issues: I began using high-tech equipment to measure their metabolisms. Over the following months, I had my patients wear a mask that measured their breath to determine what their metabolic rate was before and after meals, how it was affected by one food versus another, and what it was before, during, and after exercise. I thought this method would allow me to fine-tune the "calories in, calories out" formula—that in matching my approach to each patient's specific test results, I could be more accurate than the textbook calculations I had previously used. Based on this strategy, I drafted individual eating and exercise plans calculated to effect weight loss in each patient.

WEIGHT LOSS 2.0 FAILS

To my surprise and dismay, though I had perfected the "calories in, calories out" equation, tailoring it to each patient based on their individual metabolic tests, the new results were no better than the previous results. Patients who did respond to my treatment plan only kept the weight off temporarily. Patients could eat all the "right" foods and exercise "correctly" and still have trouble losing their excess weight, maintaining the weight they lost, or keeping their weight from increasing. In spite of all the science and technology I had at my fingertips, I could not get my patients' bodies to respond in any meaningful way.

THE UNLIKELY ANOREXIA CONNECTION

As I analyzed my overweight and obese patients' metabolisms and blood work, I noticed striking similarities to those of my anorexic patients. I realized that obese patients and anorexic patients, including those who were severely underweight, had far more in common metabolically than most people would ever suspect. Their blood work showed that both their bodies thought they were starving. How could someone's overweight body feel it was as starving as someone's underweight body? I first suspected that my overweight patients' low-calorie and low-carb dieting history had caused this confusion in their body—but over time I learned that it was more complicated than that.

BETTER SCIENCE

I thought I was being so scientific in measuring metabolism to find the right formula for weight loss, but it turned out I was not being scientific enough. As I looked at all the data, I realized that the "calories in, calories out" solution to weight management is ancient history (it was first popularized between 1910 and 1930) and terribly inadequate. It was with great relief that I finally found a treasure trove of science that explained what really drives weight problems. I began to challenge antiquated assumptions and embrace a purely scientific perspective—one that would finally allow my patients to begin to navigate their weight problems in an effective way.

Today, the majority of patients I treat in my clinical practice at Seattle Performance Medicine have experienced significant improvements in their health, metabolism, and weight by applying a scientific approach rather than by dieting and engaging in extreme exercise.

THERE'S HOPE

In this book, I will explain to you why diet and exercise are not a cure for weight problems, and I will explain the complex science of overweight and obesity in a way that's easy to understand. You'll learn why obesity is actually caused by a medical condition—not a behavioral problem, as many would have you believe—and how weight and health are not the same thing.

Next, I'll introduce you to hormones and how they communicate with the brain to control your body weight.

We'll delve into common problems that affect the metabolism, appetite, and weight, and I'll explain how these problems add up to what I call the Metabolic Storm™, where the information feedback loop between your body and brain that keeps weight in balance is thrown off and malfunctions. We'll also talk about typical hormonal imbalances that lead to weight problems and their symptoms. Along the way, I'll share stories and comments from patients who have faced these struggles and experienced these symptoms.[1]

I will present scientific evidence in the following pages that diets slow the metabolism down, something I call Diet Fog™. You will learn that weight regain after dieting is not the result of having stopped dieting, but rather a result of the fact that the diets stop working as Diet Fog sets in. We'll discuss how dieting can precipitate an acceleration of metabolic disturbance—so much so that it can sometimes cause the Metabolic Storm to escalate to a Category 5 hurricane. And finally, I will introduce you to promising new inventions that can help calm the Metabolic Storm for the majority of people, making future obesity treatment better for everyone.

In understanding how the metabolism controls weight, you'll come to understand why diets don't work long-term.

---

1. All patients have given consent to publish their stories and comments. Their names have been changed to protect their privacy.

You don't fail at dieting; it's the diets that fail you. And today's science offers great hope. As one of my patients said so succinctly, "I always knew there was science. I always believed there was a physiological explanation."

Finally, all of us deserve to know that weight problems are not our fault. All of us—including you.

CHAPTER 1

Fat Prejudice:
The Last Acceptable Bias

OVER THE PAST ONE HUNDRED years, scientists have discovered numerous hormones that are involved in weight regulation. We now have at our fingertips an enormous body of published scientific research describing the millions of chemical reactions that take place in the body and are collectively responsible for controlling body weight, metabolism, and appetite.

In spite of all this scientific knowledge, there is no current consensus among physicians or insurers in the U.S. about whether overweight and obesity even *are* a medical problem. Like the general public, many healthcare providers believe weight issues are caused by behavioral or emotional problems, a theory that was first heavily promoted in the 1950s.

Recently, however, even the conservative American Medical Association (AMA) announced that it voted to classify obesity as a disease. In doing so, the AMA joins The American Society for Metabolic and Bariatric Surgery (ASMBS), The Obesity Society (TOS), The American Society of Bariatric Physicians (ASBP), and the American Association of Clinical Endocrinologists (AACE) in regarding obesity as a disease.

This viewpoint is still far from universal, but regardless of their position on whether weight difficulties are a medical or a behavioral/emotional problem, everyone agrees on one thing: we are facing an obesity epidemic in the U.S. today.

Consider this: if overweight and obesity were caused by behavioral or emotional problems it would mean that the 30 percent of the U.S. population who are in the normal weight range are the only people in the country who are in control of their behavior. This isn't logical, of course. Or true.

There is another explanation: biological factors, not behavioral flaws, are the root cause of weight problems. Since the early 1900s, but especially in the last two decades, researchers have made incredible discoveries related to the intricacies of weight and metabolism regulation. Admittedly, the science of metabolism and weight regulation is very complex; as a student of the topic, I can attest to that. However, it's absolutely worth taking the time to learn about the basics, especially if you or your loved ones belong to the nearly 70 percent of people in the U.S. who are overweight or obese.

BMI: FULL OF FLAWS

Overweight and obesity are commonly measured by BMI (Body Mass Index). BMI, created in the 1800s by a statistician, is a mathematical formula that determines the ratio of a person's height to weight. But the formula applies the same way to everyone—whether you are male, female, young, old, athletic, sedentary, or have a large or small bone frame—and, in many cases, this one-size-fits-all method of measuring what constitutes a normal weight is an inaccurate indication of health and body fat. Muscular men and large-boned women invariably fall into the "overweight" or "obese" BMI categories, even when they do not have excess body fat.

There are other ways to define obesity, such as by measuring the amount of body fat on an individual or by analyzing the *location* of their body fat—for example, focusing on visceral fat (around organs). These measurements are much more accurate than the often misleading BMI formula.

BEING OVERWEIGHT IS NO PICNIC

Many of my overweight patients report a variety of symptoms, including in some cases, preoccupation with food, feeling hungry all the time, not feeling satisfied after eating, or knee pain, fatigue, and body aches.

Jane, for example, who had struggled with obesity since her twenties, was at her wit's end when she came to see me. A large amount of fat hung beneath her arms, making them feel so heavy that she was having trouble lifting them. "I feel like I have dumbbells attached to my arms!" she lamented. "It's miserable!"

Activities that others take for granted require a lot more physical work for people who carry extra weight. Daniel, who started dieting as a young boy, is now an amazing cyclist. When I tested his fitness, he was able to push as much power as competitive elite cyclists. His fitness level was right up there with those who finish toward the front of the pack at cycling races. But, because Daniel carries an extra one hundred pounds, a large part of his energy is dedicated to moving his body against gravity. So despite the fact that he's more fit than most of his competitors, he finishes in the back of the pack in every

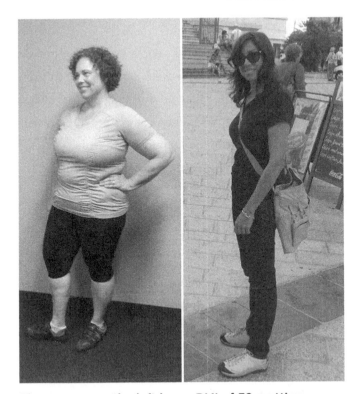

The woman on the left has a BMI of 38, putting her in the obese category. In spite of her excess weight, her measured fitness level falls in the "very fit" category. The fitness level of the woman on the right, who is in the normal-weight category, falls in the "unfit" category.

event. No one who watched him compete would ever realize he's actually stronger than most of the group. This is why fitness cannot be accurately judged by BMI or by who finishes first. When I told Cheryl her weight problem was the result of a medical problem, she said, "I can't tell you how often I've heard people say that my weight issues just boil down to how weak I am. I have to show I'm extra 'whatever' to make up for being fat. I've always had to organize my personality around proving myself." Yet another example of the many ways in which society's view of excess weight interferes with quality of life.

WEIGHT IS NOT THE PROBLEM, IT'S A SYMPTOM

Tom weighs more than 450 pounds. When he came to see me, he was looking for help getting his weight down. Everyone is worried that he's going to have a stroke or a heart attack any minute. When I tested Tom, however, not only was his blood pressure in the optimal part of the normal range but his cholesterol levels were, too.

Some overweight or obese people do develop chronic diseases such as diabetes, hypertension, heart disease, kidney failure, and some cancers. We often hear that carrying excess weight increases the risk of developing these and other diseases. But the science of obesity challenges that theory by pointing out that excess weight, high blood pressure, high blood sugar, and high cholesterol or triglycerides are frequently identified as symptoms of an underlying problem with a common root cause. Weight, therefore, is a symptom of an underlying problem, but not necessarily the cause of many associated health concerns. In fact, researchers have found that 51 percent of overweight and 32 percent of obese patients are healthy in terms of blood pressure, cholesterol, and blood glucose levels.[1]

Sean weighs 165 pounds. When he came to see me, he was confused about why, in spite of years of experience as a rock climber and mountaineer, he couldn't improve his fitness. From the outside, one would judge Sean to be the picture of health. When I tested him, however, I found that his blood pressure was elevated, his heart arteries were filled with plaque, and he had pre-diabetes. We often assume that maintaining a normal weight is a sign of health, but in reality scientists have found that 24 percent of normal-weight people have chronic diseases that are often attributed only to people who are obese.

I will explain in the coming chapters how excess weight is a symptom of a metabolism that isn't functioning normally, and how the underlying metabolic malfunctions that cause weight gain can, in some cases, trigger other medical conditions and diseases, such as high blood

1. R.P. Wildman, P. Muntner, K. Reynolds, et al., "The Obese Without Cardiometabolic Risk Factor Clustering and the Normal Weight With Cardiometabolic Risk Factor Clustering: Prevalence and Correlates of 2 Phenotypes Among the U.S. Population (NHANES 1999-2004)," *Archives of Internal Medicine* (August 11, 2008), 168(15), doi: 10.1001/ archinte.168.15.1617: 1617-1624.

pressure, cholesterol problems, and diabetes. A weight problem is merely a visible sign of hidden metabolic disease—not the cause of poor health.

THE DIABESITY EPIDEMIC

We are faced with a global obesity epidemic today, and the U.S. is in the top tier of countries affected. According to the Centers for Disease Control and Prevention (CDC), just under 70 percent of U.S. adults[2] were either overweight or obese in 2010. They also found that more than one-third of American children and adolescents were overweight and almost 20 percent were obese.[3] This means that, according to the most recent data available, only about 30 percent of American adults and less than half of children are a normal weight. In addition to obesity trends climbing, experts project that by the year 2020 about 60 percent of the U.S. adult population will have either pre-diabetes or diabetes.[4] This combined epidemic

---

2. "Obesity and Overweight," *Faststats*, http://www.cdc.gov/nchs/fastats/overwt.htm.

3. "Childhood Obesity Facts," *Centers for Disease Control and Prevention*, http://www.cdc.gov/healthyyouth/obesity/facts.htm

4. M.D. Huffman, S. Capewell, H. Ning, et al., "Cardiovascular health behavior and health factor changes (1988-2008) and projections to 2020: Results from the National Health and Nutrition Examination Surveys," *AHA Circulation*, (May 2012), 125(21): 2595-2602.

of diabetes and obesity is often referred to as the Diabesity Epidemic.

Keith, a fourth-year medical student who rotated through my office, enjoyed working with our patients who were trying to get to the bottom of their weight-loss resistance. He spent much of his time at my practice learning about metabolism and how to diagnose patients with "pre-pre-diabetes" (insulin resistance).

Just as Keith was getting ready to move on to his residency program at a major university, he worried, "I won't be allowed to run these tests on my patients, will I?" Since obesity is not universally considered a treatable disease, the medical establishment and insurance companies theoretically have no justification for running tests to diagnose the underlying causes of obesity. As opposed to proactive, preventive medicine, where diagnosis and treatment are applied before a condition develops, the current medical philosophy in the U.S. is based on reactive treatment and short-term cost containment.

For example, health providers do not routinely run tests to diagnose insulin resistance. It is not until insulin resistance progresses to diabetes that diagnosis and treatment are considered necessary. An insulin-resistant patient, Carmen, told me recently that her previous doctor said a behavioral program was her only recourse for weight loss—there was nothing else he could do for her until she developed diabetes.

Many preventive tests are considered unnecessary because of our medical system's myopic focus on cost containment. When I was asked to evaluate Keith after his rotation, one of the top criteria for rating his expertise and performance was his demonstration of being "conscious of cost containment." According to the evaluation's rating scale of one to five, Keith could only receive a top score of five if he showed expertise in saving money.

Not only was Keith judged by more than his medical skills during his training, he was not taught about obesity as a disease in medical school. He told me that there was barely a mention of insulin resistance in his medical school textbooks and that he found only one paragraph about pre-diabetes in them as well. I checked for myself and found that the typical textbook used in medical school, Current Medical Diagnosis & Treatment, is more than 1,700 pages long but dedicates only nine pages to diabetes and six pages to obesity. What's worse, one of the primary texts used in residency after medical school for doctors-in-training, Harrison's Principles of Internal Medicine—more than 3,500 pages long—devotes only 35 pages to diabetes and 14 pages to obesity, but includes 20 pages on terrorism and clinical medicine. Believe me, I want everyone to be safe. It's important. But should that subject really be given more attention than something that affects up to 70 percent of the U.S. population? In my twenty-five-year career, I've never witnessed a case of bioterrorism—but every day I see several patients who are affected by pre-diabetes, diabetes, or obesity.

Health experts predict that the Diabesity Epidemic will affect 60 percent of adults in the U.S. within the next five to ten years, yet the doctors who will care for these affected people in the near future are not receiving adequate training to diagnose and treat obesity as a disease. In the long run, our lack of attention to this problem, especially in medical schools and residency training programs, will serve only to contribute to the epidemic's growth.

WHO'S HEALTHIER?

In addition to the myth that diets solve weight problems long-term, "weight" and "health" have long been conflated and confused by popular culture. The truth is, many people of high body weight are healthy, and many are fit. The public perception is usually that weight and health are one and the same—that if you are thin you are healthier and more fit than someone who is overweight. However, science actually suggests that once we reach a certain age we are healthier when we are at the top of the normal range or in the overweight range than we are when we're in the lower part of the normal range or in the underweight range.[5] Statistics show that normal-weight

---

5. V. Hughes, "The big fat truth," *Nature*, May 2013.

people do live longer than both extremely underweight and extremely obese people. But you may be surprised to learn who lives longest of all: overweight people![6]

WEIGHT AS A STIGMA

Despite all the groundbreaking scientific discoveries that have been made over the past two decades regarding the metabolic basis of obesity, research shows that weight discrimination is still as prevalent today as race discrimination, and that many people believe weight stigma is justified and can actually motivate people to lose weight.[7]

"I experienced unbelievable harassment at work from co-workers, to the point where I was uncomfortable eating around anybody," said one of my patients, who is a highly skilled nurse. "They would say, 'Fat people are lazy,' that we have no willpower. They would sit there and be talking about overweight people as though I were not even there. Ironically, I'm a very hard worker and can stick

---

6. Kaiser Permanente Center for Health Research, *Underweight and Extremely Obese Die Earlier than People of Normal Weight, Study Finds,* at http://www.kpchr.org/research/public/News.aspx?NewsID=35 (June 23, 2009).

7. R.M. Puhl, C.A. Heuer, "Obesity Stigma: Important Considerations for Public Health," *American Journal of Public Health* (June 2010), Vol. 100, No. 6: 1019.

to something until it's done. I get a lot done on my to-do list, which takes a lot of willpower, right?"

I can't tell you how many patients have sat in my office in tears over offensive comments from a family member, friend, co-worker, or, yes, healthcare provider who was trying to be "helpful."

"Fat equates to being lazy and undisciplined; I know that's what people think," Kate, whom you will learn more about in the following chapters, said. "It hurts me because I know I'm not undisciplined. I know that I'm strong mentally and I have strong discipline. It feels like my body has betrayed me. Everything I put in my mouth turns straight to fat. But no one wants to listen to me, so I don't even try."

Although she told her doctor that she was training for an Ironman and still gaining weight, Kate said, "My doctor said, 'Honestly, I think that sometimes you just gotta buck up!'"

One of my patients, Amanda, told me about a terrible experience she had with an orthopedic surgeon recently. She had been trying hard to lose weight, participating in an intensive, boot camp-style diet and exercise program— and she suffered a hip injury in the course of the program. When she saw the orthopedist, he told her that she needed surgery but wasn't a candidate because she was "too big for the instruments."

Amanda, of course, was shocked.

"If you want surgery," the orthopedist then proceeded to say, "you need to lose weight. It's just calories in, calories out. It's a basic formula." To add insult to injury, the office walls were covered with photographs of the lean, fit orthopedist participating in triathlons. Amanda said it felt as if the photographs were saying, "I'm better than you."

Researchers have reported that fat prejudice is rampant among healthcare professionals. "Basically, my past medical providers said, 'You can't possibly be eating that much and exercising that much and not losing any weight; it's not physically possible,'" recalled one of my patients. "Put down the fork," another person's doctor urged. What is said to children is possibly the most concerning and damaging: "You really have to stop eating the cookies," or "You should lay off the computer games"—even when the child is not engaging in any of these behaviors.

Studies show that many nurses describe obese patients in negative terms and report that they tend to spend less time with someone obese than they do with a normal-weight patient. In a study led by a Yale University psychologist, 35 to 48 percent of nurses said they feel uncomfortable caring for obese people, and 31 to 42 percent said they'd rather not care for them at all.[8]

---

8. M.B. Schwartz, et al. "Weight Bias among Health Professionals Specializing in Obesity," *Obesity Research* (September 2003), Vol. 11, No. 9.

Even obesity specialists demonstrate bias. The Yale study found that the stigma against people with weight problems is so strong that many people who study and treat obesity—people who understand that obesity is caused by a combination of genetic and environmental factors—believe that overweight people are lazy, stupid, and worthless. No wonder many people with weight problems avoid going to the doctor.

"If I have a cold, somehow it's due to my weight," one of my patients once told me. "If I have a sports-induced back sprain, it's most certainly thought to be due to my weight. No matter what my health issue, my doctors tend to blame my weight."

Many of my patients have reported that their experiences with healthcare providers have frequently been frustrating and disheartening. And despite the vast body of science that suggests otherwise, excess weight is still usually not viewed as a medical problem but rather as a behavioral or emotional one, which means that patients are often left dealing with their health problems on their own.

BREAKING THE SPELL

The science of metabolism is very complicated, and it's up against a tremendous amount of discrimination, stigma, and widely dispersed misinformation. In the following chapters, you may read things that seem contrary to what you've heard before. I am going to tell you about fascinating new discoveries and inventions, and share the hope they provide today and will provide in the future. Once you understand what is really going on inside your brain and body, I'm sure you will realize that being overweight or obese cannot possibly be your fault.

CHAPTER 2

The Diet Myth

ALTHOUGH MOST PEOPLE—and even mainstream medicine—believe dieting is the only answer to weight loss, science demonstrates that there are more promising ways to deal with obesity. Dieting is not the only answer— in fact, it's not the answer at all. Diets may bring short-term success, but in the long run they nearly always fail.

For many, dieting starts at a very young age. Many of my adult patients describe a childhood of locked cabinets and refrigerators, food hidden from sight, endless visits to the doctor or weight-loss clinics, even counting calories before they were fifteen years old. For others, however, it begins later in life—either after a gradual or sudden weight gain.

I'd like to share my patient Kate's story with you. Like many of my patients, she was labeled "chubby" when she was a young girl, and she dieted for much of her life, beginning at age eleven. In spite of trying one diet after another, year after year, Kate could never get to her goal weight. Instead, she gained and lost the same five to fifteen pounds over and over again. "Diets never really worked for me," Kate recalled. This went on through her twenties and thirties until she finally gave up on dieting—at least for a while.

IT ALL COMES OFF

This changed when Kate, by now significantly overweight, became fed up with her situation and decided to give her all to a program at her fitness club. Throughout the fifteen-month program, she meticulously adhered to a low-calorie diet and diligently kept up regular aerobic exercise. Through her persistent efforts, she lost eighty-five pounds and landed in a normal weight range. She was ecstatic. "I thought I had found the magic key to my weight problem," she said.

ATHLETE AT THE STARTING LINE

Kate maintained her new, lower weight for about two years, remaining careful about her dietary choices and portion sizes and exercising regularly. She had never been athletic before, but she realized that after two years of consistently working out she was fit and strong, and she enjoyed every aspect of exercise and fitness. "I wanted to run marathons," Kate said, "but my trainer suggested triathlons to protect my knees. Little did he know I would eventually participate in Ironman competitions, which include not only the marathons that I really wanted to run but a 2.4-mile swim and a 112-mile bike ride *on top of* the marathon (26.2 miles), all in a continuous, one-day event!"

Like most Ironman athletes, as Kate ramped up her training she began to do fifteen to twenty hours of exercise per week, including workouts in all three sports: swimming, biking, and running. Many days included "brick" workouts, which are bike rides followed back-to-back by a run, or a swim followed immediately by a bike ride. Some days were double workout days: one in the morning and another in the afternoon.

TANKING UP? OR RUNNING ON FUMES?

Kate's Ironman workouts were meant to improve her endurance fitness. They burned about 500 calories per hour—which, since she was working out so much, translated to up to 10,000 calories per week. Someone

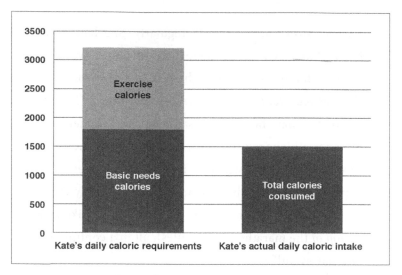

Kate was eating only 1,500 calories a day—less than half of the 3,228 calories needed to fuel her basic daily needs and twenty hours of exercise a week.

her size usually needs around 1,800 calories a day just for day-to-day activities like dressing, showering, and going to work.

When it came to her training nutrition plan, Kate used the same basic strategy that had helped her lose eighty-five pounds: portion control, low-carb intake (though she allowed herself a little more carbs than before), low fat intake, and high protein intake. She continued to count calories as meticulously as she had while losing weight and during the past years of maintenance. She increased her daily calorie intake to support her exercise—but only by 300 calories—from 1,200 to 1,500 calories.

If we do the math, Kate was eating only half of the calories per day that she needed to support her body size and workout schedule. She didn't realize that this new regimen actually represented a more extreme diet than she had ever been on before.

WHERE DID THE MAGIC GO?

Although this will be unfathomable to most people, Kate regained more than three quarters of the weight she had lost (sixty-five pounds) while training nearly twenty hours per week and consuming only 1,500 calories per day. She was devastated.

"At first I thought it was muscle, but more and more pounds kept coming on, and I got slower and slower," lamented Kate, who was participating in at least twelve triathlons each year at the time as part of her training.

"I kept trying to drop the weight, but it wasn't coming off, and worse, it was increasing steadily—even when I used the same methods I'd used to lose the original eighty-five pounds! I felt like I was stuck between a rock and a hard place. I asked myself, 'Where do I go from here? I can't eat less and I can't exercise more. So what do I do?'"

WAKING THE SLEEPING TIGER

By the time Kate came to my office, she was completely frustrated and confused about what was going on.

"How did this happen?" she sobbed.

Like many patients struggling with their weight, we soon discovered that Kate had an undiagnosed medical problem that had caused her weight struggles since childhood—and it was a problem that diet and exercise could not cure. When she exercised so much while consuming a limited diet, Kate's condition caused her body to perceive her well-meaning tactics as deprivation, and this activated a powerful weight defense system that made her body store all her fuel as fat for protection.

Like most people, Kate did not know that the body could carry so much extra fat and still feel deprived. When she found out that this was what was happening, she was stunned: "It just doesn't seem possible that you can diet and exercise your way to *more* weight. You are doing everything that people say will work, and it doesn't!"

THE DEEPER TRUTH

Everywhere we turn we hear, "Eat less and exercise more if you want to lose weight." People with higher body weight get this advice from well-meaning friends, co-workers, family members, athletic trainers, and healthcare provid-

JUST THE FACTS

It is estimated that there are 75-100 million dieters in the U.S. and the typical American dieter now makes four weight loss attempts per year.

ers. However, at least sixty years of scientific research has consistently shown that while diets do cause short-term weight loss, they don't produce significant or permanent long-term results in most overweight and obese people. And although every textbook on obesity clearly states this fact, very few people are aware of it. If diet and exercise didn't work for Kate, who was training nearly twenty hours per week and competing in Ironman events, what hope is there for everyone else? What better way to illustrate what science has been telling us for decades than with her story?

DIET SPORT

Dieting is a popular activity in the U.S., even among people of normal body weight. So many people—young and old, male and female, athletic and sedentary—are dieting. It's practically a hobby or a sport at this point. I always ask my patients who've never had a weight problem *why* they are dieting. The response is usually, "My friend was doing it, so I thought I'd try too," or, "Several of my co-workers recommended it." In our society, thinner is promoted as being better. No matter what someone weighs, they think they should weigh less.

NO HARM DONE, RIGHT? WRONG.

Scientific evidence proving that dieting rarely solves weight problems in the long term has long existed, but there's something else interesting about dieting: over the past sixty years, scientists have found that rather than helping with weight loss, diets can actually promote future weight *gain* because of their impact on metabolism. Almost all of my patients have experienced this devastating side effect of dieting, but until they came to see me, many of them had never before realized that the diet itself—which they viewed as successful in the short term—was what provoked their eventual weight gain.

Consider this common scenario: A sixteen-year-old girl of normal body weight goes on her first crash diet wanting to lose ten pounds to fit into a smaller sized junior prom dress. She successfully loses the weight in time for the prom, but afterwards begins to slowly regain the lost weight—and a then a little bit more. At seventeen, she goes on another diet and loses weight again, only to gradually regain the lost weight, plus even more. At twenty-

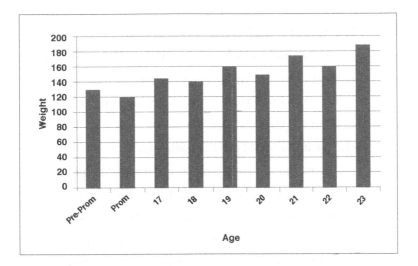

Dieting provoked weight gain in this young woman, who never had a weight problem before she dieted.

five, the young woman, who never had a weight problem before her first diet, now weighs almost 200 pounds.

Scientists have found that dieting, especially for a child or adolescent, is associated with a higher rate of obesity in adulthood than it is for non-dieters. When normal-weight people repeatedly diet, sooner or later they are likely to trigger a metabolic problem, particularly if they are genetically inclined to have one. More often than not, they eventually find themselves seriously overweight and boxed into a corner because their diets stop working, even in the short term.

THE CALM BEFORE THE STORM

Most of my patients whose weight was elevated *before* their first diet have an underlying problem that hijacks the complex system that controls their metabolism. This chaotic disruption, which affects metabolism, weight, and appetite, is what I call the Metabolic Storm.

Dieting initially leads to a temporary shift in metabolism, which makes it seem at first like things are going very well. The appetite is calmer, weight is coming off, and energy levels are improving. As Kate said, it feels like you've found the "magic key" to your weight problems. But when a person has underlying metabolic problems, the body doesn't accurately perceive the excess weight or the food supply, and it begins to panic.

FOG SETS IN

Even when a diet gets off to a good start, before long the brain detects deprivation, and it interprets it as starvation. Even in overweight patients, the brain "sees" only the current deprivation triggered by dieting—it's blind to the excess weight, so it tells the body to store fat for protection.

This is the turning point—the moment in which the body stops letting go of excess weight. I call this deprivation detection and weight-loss reversal Diet Fog. Once deprivation is detected, the body's weight defense system activates. As Diet Fog thickens, weight loss halts and gradually begins to reverse. Furthermore, Diet Fog slows the metabolism by a different mechanism than that of the original underlying metabolic problem, masking the root malfunction and making it harder for a physician to detect.

POURING GASOLINE ON THE FIRE

Over time, the metabolic irregularities caused by chronic dieting and the underlying medical issues that were originally impacting weight compound one another, catapulting people's weight higher than it was before they dieted. This uncontrollable weight rebound, which is often accompanied by constant hunger and reduced satiety, can cause individuals to revert to, and even surpass, their initial, pre-diet weight. As their weight increases uncontrollably, patients become extremely distressed, especially because they worked so hard to lose the weight in the first place. But the more they try to lose weight, the more they gain. Their chronic Metabolic Storm has now become a raging, Category 5 hurricane.

Although diets may at first seem successful, scientists have found that by five years after starting a diet most people will have regained all the weight they lost—and a high percentage of those people will weigh *more than* their pre-diet weight.[1]

THE TRUTH IS OUT THERE

Although you would never guess, based on the messages routinely promoted by the diet industry, the media, and even healthcare providers, the scientific research showing that diets are not effective long-term solutions is not only widely available in medical and scientific journals but also in every specialized advanced textbook written on the subject of obesity.

A study published in the *International Journal of Obesity*[2] in 2010, for example, examined the long-term weight-loss maintenance of 14,306 adults ages 20 to 84 who participated in the National Health and Nutrition Examination Survey (NHANES). NHANES is a series of interviews and physical exams that the National Center for Health Statistics has conducted since 1971 to gauge

---

1. T. Mann, A. J. Tomiyama, E. Westling, A. Lew, B. Samuels, J. Chatman, "Medicare's Search for Effective Obesity Treatments: Diets Are Not the Answer," *American Psychologist* (April 2007), Vol. 62, No. 3, doi: 10.1037/0003-066X.62.3.220: 220–233.

2. J. L. Kraschnewski, J. Boan, J. Esposito, et al., "Long-term weight loss maintenance in the United States," *International Journal of Obesity* (May 18, 2010), 34, doi:10.1038/ijo.2010.94: 1644–1654.

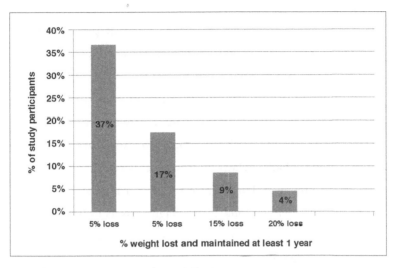

The 2010 NHANES found that over a one-year period, only 37% of participants maintained a 5% weight loss; 17% a 10% weight loss; 9% a 15% weight loss; and 4% a 20% weight loss.

the American public's health and nutritional status. The researchers discovered that among people who had been overweight or obese at some point in their life, 37 percent had maintained at least a five percent weight loss, 17 percent had maintained at least a 10 percent weight loss, 9 percent had maintained at least a 15 percent weight loss, and 4 percent reported keeping off at least a 20 percent weight loss for one year.

These results were reported as good news. The study concluded that one in six people maintained a weight loss of at least 10 percent in the long term (their definition of "long term" was at least one year), a higher percentage of long-term weight maintenance than researchers previously believed possible.

But let's take a closer look. The people who reported losing the greatest amount of weight were the least likely to keep the weight off. Even people who lost 5 percent of their weight had a relatively low success rate in weight-loss maintenance. Furthermore, there's a big catch: The researchers defined long-term weight loss as lasting one year or more. When someone has spent much of their life overweight or obese, a year is a very short time. Yes, most overweight people would love to lose even just 5 percent of their body weight, but they also want to keep that weight off—and most fail to do so.

Let's consider two hypothetical people: Mary, who at 5'4" weighs 200 pounds, and Walter, who at 5'10" weighs 300. Mary's BMI is 35, placing her in the "obese" category. Walter's BMI is 43, placing him in the "extremely obese" category.

Mary and Walter go on a diet to lose weight. The research shows that the odds are somewhat good (37 percent) that each will maintain a five percent weight loss for a year or more. This equates to ten pounds for Mary, bringing her to 190 pounds, and fifteen pounds for Walter, bringing him to 285 pounds.

The odds are less than half as good (17 percent) that they'll maintain the 10 percent weight loss that would

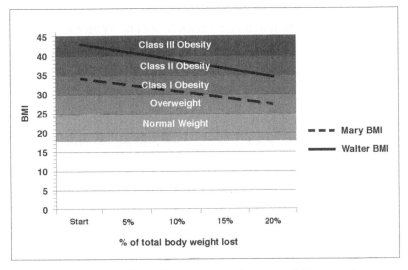

In spite of only a 4% success rate, even if Mary and Walter were somehow able to lose twenty percent of their original body weight and maintain that weight loss, neither would have lost enough weight to reach the "normal weight" BMI range.

bring Mary's weight to 180 (a 20-pound loss) and Walter's to 270 (a 30-pound loss). And if either wants to maintain a 15 percent weight loss, their chances of doing so drop almost in half again, to 9 percent—but if successful, Mary would weigh 170 pounds (a thirty-pound loss) and Walter 255 pounds (a forty-five-pound loss).

At 4 percent, the odds are slim that either will maintain a 20 percent weight loss, which would bring Mary down to 160 pounds (a forty-pound loss) and Walter down to 240 pounds (a sixty-pound loss).

It should be noted that if both Mary and Walter were able to lose 20 percent of their original body weight, Mary's BMI would still be in the overweight category and Walter's BMI would still be in the obese category. In spite of all their hard work and a slim chance of maintaining their weight loss, neither would have reached the normal weight category.

Another study published in the *International Journal of Obesity*[3] in 2005 found that whether study participants only dieted or dieted and exercised at the same time, by the one-year mark they had regained about 50 percent of their initial weight loss. The people who only dieted lost twenty-two pounds on average, while those who dieted and exercised lost an average of 29 pounds. Yet for all their hard work and great initial results, by the end of one year the people who only dieted regained ten of their twenty-two pounds lost, and those who dieted and exercised regained fifteen of their twenty-nine pounds lost. And if they gained this much back before the end of the first year, what is to stop all the weight from coming back?

---

3. C.C. Curioni, P.M. Lourenço, "Long-term weight loss after diet and exercise: a systematic review," *International Journal of Obesity* (May 31 2005), 29, doi:10.1038/sj.ijo.0803015: 1168–1174.

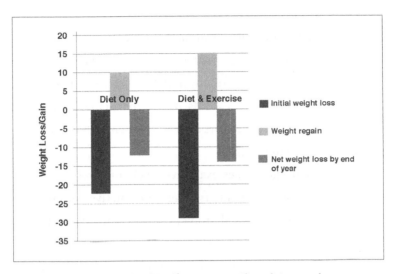

A study published in the *International Journal of Obesity* in 2005 found that whether study participants dieted or dieted and exercised at the same time, by the one-year mark they had regained about 50 percent of their initial weight lost.

THE TRUTH BEHIND THE NUMBERS

In a study published in the journal *American Psychologist*[4] in 2007, researchers from UCLA set out to identify which obesity interventions should be funded under revised Medicare guidelines that cover only obesity treatments whose effectiveness has been proven. They looked

---

4. T. Mann, A.J. Tomiyama, E. Westling, et al., "Medicare's search for effective obesity treatments: diets are not the answer," *American Psychologist* (April 2007), 62(3): 220-233.

at fourteen studies that examined calorie restrictive diets' long-term results (defined as being up to five years). The UCLA researchers discovered that, conservatively, "from one third to two thirds of diet participants will weigh *more* four to five years after the diet ends than they did before the diet began."

"Many of the studies examined likely underestimate the extent to which dieting is counterproductive because of several methodological problems, all of which bias the studies toward showing successful weight-loss maintenance," the UCLA study authors wrote. In other words, the diets studied often left people worse off, not better off. And the way the studies were designed made their results indicate that people had more success in keeping their weight off than they actually had. The authors also noted that just because a study ended and the researchers stopped following up with participants, it didn't mean that the weight gain had stopped. They noted that even in studies "with the longest follow-up times (of four or five years post-diet), the weight regain trajectories did not typically appear to level off, suggesting that if participants were followed for even longer, their weight would continue to increase."

HOW MANY DIETS HAVE YOU TRIED?

With decades of scientific research showing that dieting is a dead end for most people, you'd think that it would be out of style by now. But—understandably—people are looking for answers, and peer pressure to diet is very strong, even for normal-weight people. So for those who do suffer from weight problems, it's easy to imagine the immense pressure from family, co-workers, friends, and healthcare providers to dial up the dieting and exercise and keep "trying harder."

"I've been on thirty-two diets in my life, all prescribed by physicians," one of my patients told me. "I've been on a lifelong diet and I'm at my all-time high body weight," is another common complaint. And as one patient recently lamented, "I started dieting when I was eight, yet at fifty I'm now heavier than ever!"

WHY DO WE DO THIS TO OURSELVES?

The massive *Handbook of Obesity: Clinical Applications, Third Edition* is one of the bibles of obesity medicine. In it, Robert F. Kushner, M.D., M.S., clinical director of Northwestern University medical school's Comprehensive Center on Obesity, and Louis J. Aronne, clinical professor of medicine and director of the Comprehensive Weight-Control Program at New York-Presbyterian Hospital/ Weill Cornell Medical Center, question why patients keep trying to lose weight even though their previous attempts haven't produced long-term results. They write:

> *Given our current state of knowledge and the treatments currently available, the goal of obesity treatment should be the lowest weight the patient can comfortably maintain, which in the average patient is about 5-10% loss of total body weight. Attaining ideal body weight or a loss of 20% of body weight is not possible for the vast majority of overweight and obese people.[5]*

This means that at best, our hypothetical, 200-pound Mary would probably be able to lose only between ten and twenty pounds and keep it off, and 300-pound Walter could probably only maintain a fifteen- to thirty-pound weight loss.

Consider what University of Toronto psychologists Janet Polivy, PhD, and C. Peter Herman, PhD, both obesity researchers, write in a chapter of *Handbook of Obesity* titled "Weight Cycling as an Instance of False Hope":[6]

---

5. R.F. Kushner, L.J. Aronne, "Obesity and the Primary Care Physician," *Handbook of Obesity: Clinical Applications, Third Edition, ed.* George A. Bray and Charles Brouchard (New York, Informa, 2008), 125.

6. J. Polivy, C.P. Herman, "Weight Cycling as an Instance of False Hope," *Handbook of Obesity: Clinical Applications, Third Edition, ed.* George A. Bray and Charles Brouchard (New York: Informa, 2008), 105.

People do tend to succeed in the early stages of weight loss attempts and most dieters have at least some early success to spur them on. When weight loss slows or stops, however, people tend to become vulnerable to elements that interfere with further weight loss. The weight loss attempt is judged to have failed. Over time, however, most people experience a renewed desire to lose weight, and begin a new weight loss program or effort. This subsequent effort usually follows the same pattern.

That is to say, diets tend to work at first—at least somewhat. But over the long term, most people regain the weight and more in spite of multiple dieting attempts.

YES, EVEN THE TEXTBOOKS ARE SAYING THIS

It is bad enough to experience the heartbreak and frustration of gaining lost weight back. But what most people don't realize is that science proves that not only does dieting stand virtually no chance of working, it often makes an existing weight problem worse. Polivy and Herman continue:

Weight cycling may have metabolic effects that make subsequent weight loss efforts more difficult and contribute to subsequent obesity. Given that weight cycling appears to increase the risk of overweight/obesity, however, it seems likely that weight cycling may contribute to these problems through its ultimately elevating effect on body weight. Weight cycling thus appears to entail at least some risk, if only from the ratcheting upward of weight that seems to result from cycles of success and failure at weight loss.[7]

Translation: dieting impacts the metabolism in ways that increase the odds that people will eventually gain weight above and beyond their starting weight. As many of my patients might say, diets make you fatter.

In another important obesity medicine text, *Obesity Prevention and Treatment*, George A. Bray, MD, chief of the division of clinical obesity and metabolism at Pennington Biomedical Research Center at Louisiana State University, describes similar limitations:

---

7. J. Polivy, C.P. Herman, "Weight Cycling as an Instance of False Hope," *Handbook of Obesity: Clinical Applications, Third Edition, ed.* George A. Bray and Charles Brouchard (New York: Informa, 2008), 113.

Results from most long-term clinical studies of treatment for overweight patients show a high prevalence of weight regain. In the Institute of Medicine report "weighing the options" for those who achieved weight loss, more than one-third of the weight typically was regained within one year and nearly all within five years.[8]

Again, according to these authors it's unrealistic to expect to keep lost weight off with dieting. Whatever people lose, they're going to gain back by the end of Year Five.

It's worth noting that the report "Weighing the Options: Criteria for Evaluating Weight Management Approaches"[9] was published by a nonprofit, non-governmental health arm of the National Academy of Sciences (NAS), an organization that provides decision-makers and the public with what its website describes as "unbiased and authoritative advice." The study was published way back in 1995, when Windows was a cutting-edge

---

8. G.A. Bray, "Classification and Evaluation of the Overweight Patient," *Handbook of Obesity: Clinical Applications, Third Edition, ed.* George A. Bray and Charles Brouchard (New York: Informa, 2008), 23.

9. Committee to Develop Criteria for Evaluating the Outcomes of Approaches to Prevent and Treat Obesity, Institute of Medicine, *Weighing the Options: Criteria for Evaluating Weight Management Approaches, ed.* Paul R. Thomas (Washington, D.C.: National Academies Press, 1995).

innovation, most people were just beginning to use email, and no one had ever even heard of an iPod. Almost twenty years have passed since the study was published, and this scientific knowledge has been replicated countless times since then, yet somehow this well-established information has not broken through the massive dieting messaging in popular culture.

Of course, research like this is often buried in obscure medical publications with titles like *Clinical Obesity* and *Current Opinion in Endocrinology, Diabetes and Obesity*—not the typical publications you would download onto your Kindle, find on the newsstand, or read on the treadmill or in your doctor's waiting room.

SCIENCE NEEDS BETTER PR— WHAT'S THE HOLDUP?

It's not unusual for there to be a significant lag between when scientists make a discovery and when the medical establishment adopts the change or pharmaceutical companies invent medications that apply the new knowledge. And it takes even longer before the medications become available to the public. For example, it's not unusual for up to twenty years to pass between an important scientific discovery and the time it shows up in a medical school textbook. When it comes to metabolism discoveries, in many cases decades have passed before proven science has made its way into textbooks.

There are probably many reasons why the myth about diets' effectiveness has stuck around like gum on the bottom of a shoe. One valid rationale is that the actual science is extremely complicated. Understanding the metabolism requires a good amount of scientific knowledge and specialized study; as I mentioned in Chapter One, metabolism and weight problems are barely touched on during medical school, and once doctors are out in practice their time is limited, so many are likely to find it overwhelming to keep up with all the current research.

There are other challenges faced by the science of metabolism and obesity, of course. In 1995, an Institute of Medicine study noted that the weight-loss industry was worth billions of dollars.[10] Today, the industry is worth some $60 billion.[11] An industry with this much capital behind it has the power to give antiquated ideas tremendous weight and dissuade the American public from believing the countering science. And the weight-loss

---

10. Committee to Develop Criteria for Evaluating the Outcomes of Approaches to Prevent and Treat Obesity, Institute of Medicine, *Weighing the Options: Criteria for Evaluating Weight Management Approaches*, ed. Paul R. Thomas (Washington, D.C.: National Academies Press, 1995).

11. Brooke Axtel, "How to Be A Shameless Woman: Making Peace With Our Bodies, Ourselves," *Forbes*, September 26, 2012.

industry isn't the only industry whose existence is predicated upon this erroneous, outdated information: the media, the fitness industry, the supplements industry, book publishing, and other industries have extended these ideas' longevity as well.

We should also keep in mind that people long for an overnight fix, a miracle diet that will solve their weight problem for good. Out of desperation, they may ignore what their past experiences prove, let alone what science proves—that their diets don't work long-term, and that the weight eventually comes back in spite of all their efforts.

CHAPTER 3

Hormone Handbook: Beyond Estrogen and Testosterone

"I'VE ALWAYS DREAMED there was a problem with my metabolism that caused my body to hold on to fat," Sarah said, "but I didn't know there really WAS a problem!"

Counter to what we have all been told, weight problems really are commonly caused by metabolism problems. In this chapter, I will introduce many little-known but powerful hormones that play a major role in regulating weight, metabolism, and appetite.

BRAIN IS BOSS

Our weight, metabolism, and appetite are controlled by a complex system. The brain and body communicate in a feedback loop where the brain is the CEO and the hormones produced in the body are the messengers. These hormonal messengers provide important information about our body weight and fuel supply by using what is called the *peripheral metabolic pathway* to get their signals to the brain. Within the brain, the *central metabolic pathway* interprets those incoming signals and sends its own output signals back to the body.

WE'VE COME A LONG WAY

Over the past twenty years, many scientists have dedicated their entire career to studying these interrelated pathways. The science is complicated, but what scientists are clear about is the basic physiology of the system that regulates our metabolism, the areas where glitches can occur, the ways that we can potentially treat these glitches medically, and why diets don't work long-term. Treatments available now and those in development offer promising strategies for repairing problems along this critical pathway. New scientific research in the area of metabolism, overweight, and obesity is now progressing at such an explosive pace that it's impossible to keep up

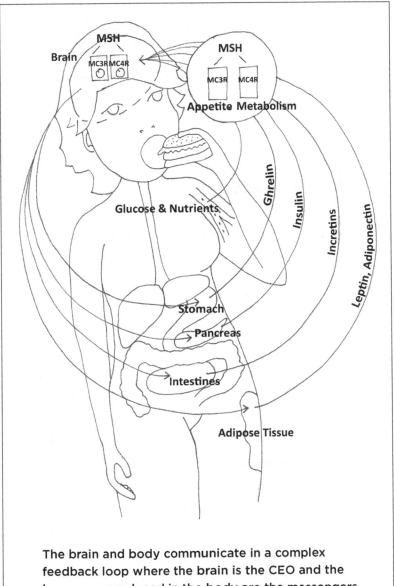

The brain and body communicate in a complex feedback loop where the brain is the CEO and the hormones produced in the body are the messengers.

with it all. As a physician treating overweight and obese patients, I have found that these fascinating new discoveries and promising inventions are already providing exciting breakthroughs for my affected patients. I cannot wait to see what the next ten years bring.

MIXED SIGNALS

My biggest breakthrough came the moment I realized that similar metabolic issues can be caused by either *perceived* underweight and malnutrition (which, interestingly, occurs in most overweight and obese patients' bodies) or *actual* underweight and malnutrition (found in underweight and anorexic patients). These two types of people have a number of common blood test results, symptoms, and physical findings. For instance, hormone levels, body temperature, satiety, and fertility may be similarly affected in overweight and anorexic patients of both sexes, and overweight female patients may even stop having regular menstrual periods, just as anorexic patients can.

I knew that science supported this finding. However, it wasn't until I finally measured and compared the labs of my overweight and underweight patients that I saw exactly how close the body's experience of perceived starvation is to actual starvation.

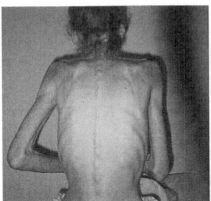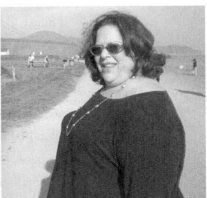

The patient on the left has a BMI of about 12 due to anorexia. The patient on the right has a BMI of about 60 due to a metabolic malfunction. These two people have common blood test results, symptoms and physical findings indicating underweight status and malnutrition (real and perceived).

The people in the photos above had similar blood levels of a neurotransmitter that signals starvation.

The metabolic feedback loop and its hormone messengers dictate the brain and body's perception of nourishment and weight. They adjust the metabolism, body weight, and appetite according to that *perception*— whether it's real or not. Faulty hormone levels or signals lead the brain and body to perceive that a person is underweight or undernourished, even if this is not true.

Susan could not understand why she couldn't lose any weight and why she actually gained weight when she lowered her food intake to only 800 calories per day. After looking at her lab work, I noted that her levels of a hormone that informs the brain of the body's fat mass were abnormally low.

"What do you mean?" Susan asked. "My brain thinks my weight is one hundred pounds lower than it really is? I would be really underweight if that were true!"

In this type of situation the individual's metabolism reacts as though she is seriously underweight and malnourished, causing the body to desperately increase body weight and appetite, attempting to counter what it erroneously thinks is a life-threatening situation. This is why diets don't work: weight problems are often the body's way of trying to protect itself. Once you understand more about how hormones function, this will become clearer.

MEET YOUR HORMONES

Endocrine tissue manufactures and secretes *hormones* into the bloodstream and the nervous system. Hormones are chemical messengers, produced by glands, that ferry information throughout the body to regulate chemical reactions. This complex network of the hormones that specifically affect metabolism is referred to as the *peripheral metabolic pathway*. It includes chemical messengers that emanate from the fat mass, bones, muscle mass, gastrointestinal (GI) tract, pancreas, liver, endocrine glands, and blood components.

When we think of hormones, we often think of estrogen and testosterone: mood swings in adolescents and athletes on steroids, or hot flashes in middle-aged women. But hormones that regulate metabolism include well-known hormones, such as insulin, and other, lesser-known hormones like adiponectin, leptin, glucagon, ghrelin, osteocalcin, oxyntomodulin, PYY, CCK, amylin, incretins such as GLP-1 and GIP, and many more. The hormone signals travel throughout the body and to the brain via this peripheral metabolic pathway, and in doing so they collectively influence our metabolism, weight, and appetite.

Every hormone communicates a very specific set of information. Imagine your body's hormones as functioning like a TV news team, where one commentator is an expert in politics, another covers the local weather, and yet another follows the latest celebrity news. Think of these reporters as being on air all day long, reporting the news and updating viewers.

Each hormone is emitted at a specific time and in a specific pattern. One might be released once a day, while another releases several times a day and still another several times an hour. Some hormones are secreted in pulses of microscopic droplets, like an IV drip. When each hormone is released, the bloodstream and nervous system carry it to receptors throughout the body whose job is to receive the hormonal signals, much like an antenna would.

The body's fat tissue, also known as fat mass, is actually the endocrine system's largest organ. Fat plays an enormously important role in regulating metabolism and influencing inflammation responses throughout the body. Collectively, the fat mass produces and secretes more hormones and bioactive chemicals, called *adipocytokines*, than any other endocrine gland. To date, scientists have identified more than eighty different influential proteins in the fat mass, including twenty-five hormones and numerous other chemical messengers.

Our fat tissue communicates with the rest of the body and the brain to regulate metabolism, appetite, and body weight—mainly by announcing its presence. When everything is functioning normally, hormones from the fat tissue tell the brain and other body parts how much we weigh, how well-nourished we are, and how our body should respond to other endocrine hormonal signals essential to managing metabolism, weight, and appetite. Before the brain and body feel safe enough to carry out many nonessential functions—reproduction, for example—they must be convinced that the body has enough fat to survive a food emergency should one occur. Many weight problems are at least partly caused by abnormalities of certain hormones from the fat tissue.

Let's examine the role that several important hormones play in helping the metabolism function. (This is just for your information—there won't be a test on the material, I promise!)

STARS OF THE HORMONE SHOW

Insulin

Discovered in 1921, *insulin* is one of the major hormones that regulates metabolism. It is produced by the pancreas, which is located in the upper abdomen. Insulin's primary roles are to inform the brain that we are adequately nourished (have fuel on board), and to help transport glucose and proteins into the body cells so they can be used as energy.

Insulin "unlocks the door" to each cell so fuel can enter. (Note, however, that there are exceptions to this process: the brain, heart, and other vital organs can access glucose directly without requiring insulin.) Insulin's presence in the bloodstream signals to the brain and body that fuel is available, and it gives the body the green light to burn fuel that is in current circulation. It is generally produced in response to either a meal or snack, though it is also produced in smaller amounts during periods without food, such as at night or between meals when the liver releases its glucose stores to keep the blood supply steady.

Insulin can be measured with a routine lab test.

Glucagon

Glucagon was discovered in 1923. As insulin transports glucose into the cells after meals, the amount of glucose remaining in the bloodstream declines, which stimulates secretion of a second hormone from the pancreas: *glucagon.* Glucagon's role is to talk to the liver, which contains a reserve of glucose in the form of *glycogen.* Glucagon signals the liver to release a small amount of glucose into the bloodstream to "top off" the body's blood sugar between meals and keep it from dipping too low. Once the liver releases its stored glucose, the pancreas responds by secreting just enough insulin to transport any extra glucose into the cells for energy.

Scientists have recently found that glucagon, like insulin, influences the brain by providing critical information the brain needs to regulate blood sugar and metabolism. Together, glucagon and insulin maintain a steady glucose level within the body at all times, which is critical to normal metabolic function, thinking, mood, and energy. This is especially important because the brain uses nearly 100 percent glucose (which comes from dietary carbohydrates) for its own energy supply.

Glucagon, like insulin, can be measured with a routine lab test.

Leptin

Discovered in 1994, *leptin* is a powerful metabolism-regulating hormone primarily produced by fat tissue. Leptin travels through the bloodstream to receptor sites in the brain, liver, pancreas, bones, and nearly every type of body tissue. In doing so, it keeps the entire body informed and updated about how much a person weighs and whether he or she is carrying sufficient body fat to freely burn fat when the body needs energy.

The leptin signal is a major influencer of metabolism in the brain. Once received by the brain, if other reassuring signals are also present, the brain permits the appetite to regulate itself and allows the metabolism to function at full throttle. In other words, leptin from the peripheral system is required in order for the body's *satiety* cues to normalize—that is, in order for a person to feel satisfied after eating a meal. It also stimulates the metabolic rate to increase and body weight to balance. Leptin's other functions are to improve bone density, support the immune system, regulate thyroid levels, and influence reproductive hormones (it strengthens fertility in both men and women). Leptin levels can be measured clinically with a routine lab test.

Adiponectin

Discovered in 1996, *adiponectin* is another important hormone that is secreted by fat cells. Adiponectin sends

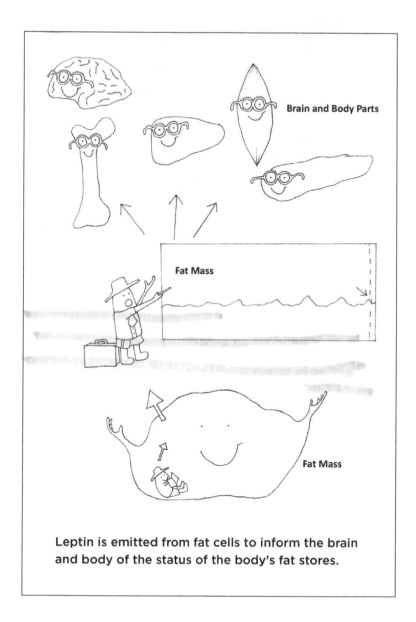

Leptin is emitted from fat cells to inform the brain and body of the status of the body's fat stores.

signals to the muscle mass, and, to a lesser degree, the brain. Adiponectin is a powerful "insulin sensitizer," meaning it increases muscle cells' sensitivity to insulin. This in turn helps insulin move glucose out of the bloodstream and into the cells more easily. Adiponectin also stimulates metabolism in the body's muscle mass at rest and during exercise and reduces total body inflammation, particularly in the blood vessels. This means that when the fat mass—the very same fat that popular culture proclaims is hazardous to good health—communicates normally, it actually plays a vital role in helping the body burn energy and in keeping blood vessels free of inflammation, which can prevent strokes, diabetes, and heart attacks.

Adiponectin levels can be measured clinically with a routine blood test.

Gut Hormones

Discovered in 1902, gut hormones are very important players in metabolism, appetite, and weight regulation. *Incretins*, which include GIP and GLP-1, are one group of hormones emitted by the gastrointestinal tract (or gut). Other gut hormones include ghrelin, PYY, oxyntomodulin, and many more.

The incretin group of gut hormones help regulate communication between the gut and the brain, telling the

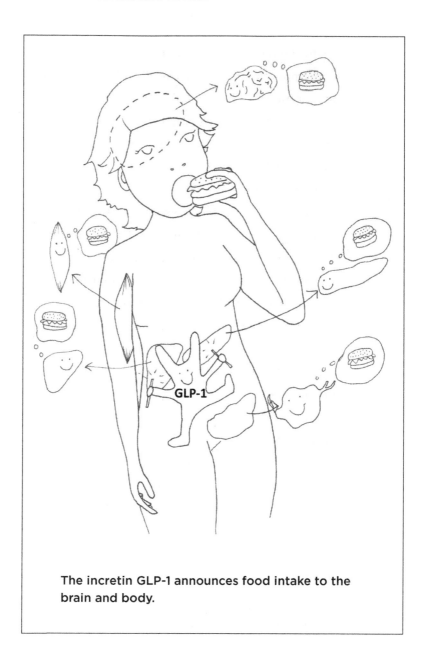

The incretin GLP-1 announces food intake to the brain and body.

JUST THE FACTS

Leptin-Adiponectin Ratio

Researchers have explored whether the ratio of leptin in the body relative to adiponectin may predict a person's risk of strokes, diabetes, heart attacks, and other catastrophic events. The higher the person's leptin level relative to the amount of adiponectin they emit, the greater, some experts believe, the person's risk is for these types of problems.

However, recent studies suggest that adiponectin levels may more accurately predict these potential health risks and hazards when measured alone, regardless of leptin levels.

brain when and what a person is eating. They control the pace at which food moves through the stomach and small intestine, and the pace at which nutrients, including glucose, are absorbed and released into the bloodstream. Incretins also help the pancreas balance insulin and glucagon levels to maintain a consistent level of glucose in the bloodstream after a person eats.

By informing and assuring the body and the brain about food availability, all the gut hormones play a major role in regulating the central metabolic pathway, appetite receptor satiety cues, and the metabolic rate. Currently, most gut hormones—including incretins—cannot be measured in a clinical setting, but many are routinely measured in research settings.

More on Ghrelin

Discovered in 1999, *ghrelin*, one of the gut hormones, is produced primarily by the tissue along the lower curve of the stomach. Ghrelin informs the brain when the body's short-term fuel supply has run out between meals and signals that food is needed.

Ghrelin is one of the few hormones that block rather than stimulate the metabolism, turning the central pathway "light" red. During ghrelin surges, metabolism slows down and appetite increases. If ghrelin fails to decline after a person eats and its baseline remains elevated, that person's weight will usually increase. Ghrelin also opposes the action of all of the hormones that turn the metabolism "on" and the appetite "down." Whereas other gut hormones (like GLP-1, oxyntomodulin, and PYY) stimulate the metabolic rate, calm the appetite receptors, and lower body weight, high ghrelin levels do the opposite.

Total ghrelin levels can be measured clinically with a routine blood test.

Amylin

Discovered in 1988, *amylin* is a hormone produced by the pancreas that helps the brain "see" the leptin signal. Therefore, it has a major role in enabling and influencing metabolic rate and satiety. Like leptin, amylin helps the brain regulate the function of the thyroid, ovaries, testicles, and several other glands. Like incretins, amylin helps regulate the pace at which nutrients empty from the stomach into the small intestine and then into the bloodstream, and it helps regulate the pancreas's glucagon response to prevent glucose levels in the blood from increasing above normal ranges.

Currently, amylin levels cannot be measured in a clinical setting, but can be measured in research settings.

THAT'S THE GANG

The hormones you've just learned about are some of the most important players along the peripheral metabolic pathway. The signals they send make their way to the brain and its central metabolic pathway, where the information is processed and acted upon.

KEY METABOLIC HORMONES & THEIR MALFUNCTIONS

Functions	Malfunctions	
Leptin	**Low Leptin**	**Leptin Resistance**
Informs brain of body weight and fat status	Decreases metabolic rate	Severely impaired satlety
Increases metabolism	Decreases reproductive and thyroid hormones	Rapid weight gain
Increases satiety	Decreases satiety	
Regulates reproductive and thyroid hormones	Increases hunger	
	Weight gain with exercise (women)	
Insulin	**Insulin Resistance**	
Informs the brain we are nourished	Weight loss resistance	
Transports glucose and protein into cells	Increases belly fat	
	Sugar cravings	
	Fatigue/low energy	
Adiponectin	**Low Adiponectin**	
Increases metabolism	Increases risk for diabetes, stroke and heart attack	
Increases insulin sensitivity	Weight loss resistance	
Anti-inflammatory	Increases inflammation	
GLP-1	**GLP-1 Malfunction**	
Informs the brain of what and when you are eating	Impairs satiety	
Controls the pace of food transport in the gut	Possible stomach bloating	
Increases satiety		
Increases metabolic rate		
Ghrelin	**High Ghrelin**	
Increases appetite	Persistent, steady weight gain (sometimes rapidly)	
Decreases satiety	Weight loss resistance	
Weight loss resistance	Sometimes excessive hunger	
Weight gain with exercise (women)		
Decreases metabolism		

METABOLIC CONDITIONS

Pre-Diabetes	Diabetes
Diagnostic criteria: HbA1C level: 5.7-6.3 Glucose level: 100-125	Diagnostic criteria: HbA1C level: 6.4+ Glucose level: 126+
Common signs and symptoms: Decreased metabolic rate	Common signs and symptoms: Decreased metabolic rate
Weight loss resistance	Weight loss resistance
Weight gain	Weight gain
Sugar cravings	Sugar cravings
Acanthosis nigricans	Acanthosis nigricans
Stretch marks	Stretch marks
Blood vessel hypertrophy	Blood vessel hypertrophy
	Increased thirst
	Increased hunger
	Frequent urination
	Changes in vision

Metabolic Syndrome
A combination of three or more of the following: Abnormal cholesterol panel such as: Increased Triglycerides Increased LDL particles Decreased HDL Increased blood pressure Increased abdominal circumference: 35" or more in women 40" or more in men Increased glucose or insulin

THE FOUR-DOOR SYSTEM

The *central metabolic pathway* is the portion of the feedback loop that consists of the brain and the nervous system. It receives incoming signals from the peripheral metabolic pathway, then processes and interprets those signals to determine whether to give a green, yellow, or red light to the body's metabolic processes. This action ultimately determines whether the body will lose, maintain, or gain weight. For simplicity's sake, I describe the central metabolic pathway as a four-door system. There are four *mandatory* doors that must open in order for the body to let go of excess weight. When glitches occur along the pathway, keeping the doors from opening normally, it can cause body fat accumulation, difficulty losing excess weight, reduced metabolism, and a heightened appetite.

Door Number One

Door One, the first door of the central metabolic pathway, is called the *arcuate nucleus* (ARC). The ARC is located within the hypothalamus, the body's highest-level gland, which governs daily operation of the body's other glands. The ARC is the entry point through which messengers coming from the peripheral metabolic pathway arrive at the brain. Here, their signals are processed.

THE "FOUR DOORS" OF
THE CENTRAL METABOLIC PATHWAY

A Normally Functioning System

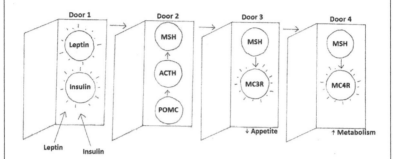

A Malfunctioning System

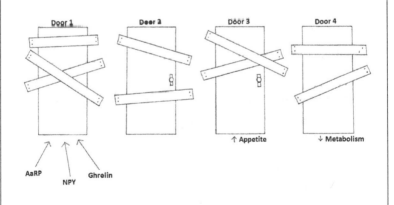

The neurons (specialized cells) within the ARC not only permeate the hypothalamus but also extend and transmit information into the next gland down in the hierarchy, the pituitary gland, which also directs other glands throughout the body.

The ARC neurons produce two chemicals—I call them "guards"—that play a major role at Door One. These chemicals are called *neuropeptide Y* (NPY), and *agouti-related protein* (AGRP). NPY and AGRP are two of the body's most powerful chemicals when it comes to blocking metabolic function. When they are elevated, they send starvation signals through the brain and body, stimulating appetite and slowing metabolism.

By default, both NPY and AGRP remain on high alert (in an elevated position), assuming that the body is in a malnourished and low body-weight state, until hormones and other messengers from the peripheral metabolic pathway successfully prove that the body weighs enough and has sufficient fuel. In other words, for our own protection, NPY and AGRP need a "coast is clear" signal to allow their levels to drop.

The problem is that, as mentioned earlier, the NPY levels of an anorexic patient with a BMI of 12 and an obese patient with a BMI over 60 can be the same even though only one of the patients is actually starving, because glitches in the feedback loop can create an erroneous perception of starvation. When NPY and AGRP remain elevated in this way, the brain thinks it's not safe to allow the metabolic process to proceed to Door Two.

Important signals are received at the ARC. Leptin signals from the body's fat tissue communicate whether a person has sufficient body mass. Insulin signals from the pancreas inform the brain that the body is in a nourished state and therefore has access to food. Glucose, GLP-1, PYY, and other messengers also send the ARC signals, providing information on nutritional status and body weight and influencing NPY and AGRP levels.

When incoming signals convince the ARC that the body has sufficient weight and nourishment, a green light is given for metabolically stimulating reactions to progress. NPY and AGRP levels are allowed to sharply decline, opening Door One and removing the obstacles to opening Door Two.

NPY can be measured clinically with a routine lab test. However, AGRP can only be measured in research settings at this time.

Door Number Two

Door Two is located in the pituitary gland. This is where the precursor hormone *propiomelanacortin* (POMC) converts to *adrenocorticotropic hormone* (ACTH), which in turn produces the metabolism-stimulating hormone *melanocyte stimulating hormone* (MSH). So, opening Door Two is really the process of converting one hormone to another: POMC to ACTH, and ACTH to MSH. Once MSH is available, there are not too many additional processes needed to allow the metabolism to increase, weight to drop, and the appetite to settle down.

However, because the body really wants to protect us in case of famine, it's not easy to open Door Two. The neurotransmitter *gamma-aminobutyric acid* (GABA) is the primary guard at this door: it puts the brakes on chemical reactions throughout the body to keep them from going too fast. A drop in NPY, however, causes GABA to drop, thus allowing Door Two to open and POMC to convert to MSH.

ACTH and MSH can be measured clinically with routine lab tests. GABA and POMC cannot be measured clinically at this time.

Door Number Three

Door Three is comprised of the *melanocortin 3 receptors* (MC3Rs) located in the hypothalamus and limbic areas (memory, motivation, and emotion centers) of the brain. MC3Rs control our appetite, affecting our interest in food and satisfaction after eating. Door Three opens when the newly formed MSH, produced from opening Door Two, connects correctly with the MC3Rs. Receptors like the MC3Rs are like antennas that receive hormone signals, in this case MSH. When the MC3Rs detects the MSH and 'opens' successfully, the body experiences normal hunger levels and feels satisfied after eating a meal. In other words, when MC3Rs work properly, people don't think about how much to eat—it's very natural and automatic.

But as in other parts of the process, there can be glitches with this step. If MSH signals are too low or if MSH has a problem connecting properly with the MC3Rs, the body is not likely to experience normal hunger and satiety cues. Instead, depending on how weak the signal is at the MC3Rs, there may be a preoccupation with food, excessive hunger, and lack of satisfaction even after a normal meal.

Genetic testing for MC3R malfunction is not yet available clinically.

Door Number Four

Door Four is comprised of the *melanocortin 4 receptors* (MC4Rs) located in the hypothalamus. MC4Rs also receive the signals from MSH. By doing so, they regulate metabolism and ultimately determine whether body weight will increase, decrease, or stay the same. Door

Four opens when MSH fits precisely into the MC4Rs. At this point, the body receives a final "all clear" signal to increase metabolic rate and reduce body weight.

However, things can go wrong at the MC4Rs. For example, if ghrelin levels are very high, or if the AGRP from Door One hasn't dropped far enough, MSH can be blocked from connecting at the MC4Rs, which means the body won't receive the green light it's waiting for.

Genetic testing for MC4R malfunction is not yet available clinically.

CHECKS AND BALANCES

The metabolic signals that flow along the central pathway in the brain communicate back to the body, relaying what the brain thinks of the body's overall nutritional status. The peripheral pathway messages, in turn, communicate back to the central pathway. If all goes smoothly, this feedback loop is a well-oiled machine. But if the feedback loop encounters a glitch, that one glitch can lead to another in a domino effect that causes higher body weight, slower metabolic function, and often appetite malfunction.

Communication between the pathways is instantaneous and dynamic. Hormones from the peripheral metabolic pathway can alter their signals, depending upon reciprocal signals from the brain. In turn the brain interprets the incoming hormonal signals and instructs the central metabolic pathway on how much fuel it should let the body burn. By communicating back and forth in this fashion, neither the brain nor the body permits the other to compromise the body's perceived nutritional status.

You might think of this communication system as being similar to the way a couple with a joint checking account might manage their account balance. A certain amount of money comes in each month, but many different ways of spending it exist: cash withdrawals, checks, online bill payments, electronic transfers, and debit or credit card purchases. Either partner (or both) can use the account simultaneously—which means that without a system of checks and balances, both partners could withdraw as much money as they wanted, with potentially disastrous consequences.

The metabolic feedback loop functions similarly, allowing each partner—in this analogy, the peripheral and central pathways—to know the account balance and make adjustments accordingly so neither partner depletes the account. The fat mass, organs, glands, receptor sites, blood components, and other elements of the peripheral system communicate to the brain and make adjustments instantaneously, preserving the energy balance they perceive as appropriate.

WRAP-UP

When leptin, insulin, and other chemical signals from the peripheral metabolic pathway convince the brain that the body is not in nutritional danger, and if no other factors interfere, the central metabolic pathway is put into motion beginning with NPY and AGRP levels dropping to open Door One. When Door One opens wide enough, usually all of the other doors open, and the metabolism is free to burn incoming fuel, body weight balances normally, and the appetite is calmed. This is what happens routinely in normal-weight people with normal metabolisms—and, as unbelievable as it may sound, when an overweight person's metabolic system has rebooted itself and starts working correctly, this will happen for them as well, and they will likely automatically begin to lose their excess weight.

As tough as it is to deal with weight problems, when glitches in the metabolic pathway occur, the body is really just doing its job: protecting us from perceived harm by storing more fat.

CHAPTER 4

Welcome to Metabolism 101

THE METABOLISM CONSISTS OF all of the biological and chemical processes that convert the food we eat into the energy our body needs to function well. The body must coordinate thousands of simultaneous metabolic activities just so the heart can beat and the brain can work.

Whether we are active or at rest, our metabolism is always hard at work managing our fuel and energy balance. Metabolism is a constant process; it may slow down or speed up, but it never stops. It is the sum total of all reactions in the body: it allows the body to convert fuel and fuel stores into energy, which, in turn, enables activities as basic as breathing and as complex as running a marathon.

Our metabolism depends on regular fuel intake to stabilize the body's nutritional status and make energy available. The body accomplishes this by following four steps: foraging (or innate eating), digestion, absorption, and finally utilization. Utilization involves converting nutrients into energy to use in one of three ways (this is called *energy partitioning*): for immediate use to power the body or brain; for later use (kept as fat stores); and for building and repairing structural body tissue like muscles, tendons, bone, and skin.

STEP 1: FORAGING—PEOPLE DO IT TOO

The first metabolic activity is *foraging*. Of course, we're familiar with animals' innate foraging behavior: bears rummage through the woods for berries, and squirrels dig for buried nuts. However, we tend to give little thought to humans having similar eating behaviors. Innate eating is not dictated by a clock or schedule; rather, it's largely driven by hormonal activity between the brain, fat, muscles, bones, gastrointestinal tract, organs, and other parts of the body that we may not even associate with our appetite.

As I mentioned in Chapter 3, the metabolism is regulated by a complex feedback loop whereby the body and the brain communicate through hormone signals. These hormones impact the appetite receptors that direct our innate eating experience. Various communication centers throughout the body inform the brain and body about the amount of food and the type of nutrients that are needed as fuel.

This inner wisdom may cause us to desire or crave foods that we innately know contain the nutrients we need in the quantities we need them. How do we know this? Because our ancestors' survival depended on knowing what nutrients certain foods contained, and their evolved eating habits have influenced our DNA.

Let's say you develop a distinct craving for tomatoes. You decide to make spaghetti with red sauce and eat it for dinner that night and as lunch the next day. If this satisfies your taste for tomatoes, you may not crave them again for a while. Maybe it's just that you knew it would taste good—but it's also possible that your body needed to obtain a specific nutrient found in tomatoes, and that's what caused you to crave them. Once you eat some tomatoes, the nutritional need is met, and your appetite for tomatoes may go away for a while.

These types of cravings can be incredibly specific. We're all familiar with stories of pregnant women who develop a taste for pickles or some other unusual food. Sometimes people even yearn for foods they've never had before. When this happens, it's likely that the brain is acting upon information that's been passed down through generations genetically.

Food as a Distraction

When the metabolism is functioning normally, food generally isn't overly attractive—a bag of chips in the cupboard or donuts at the office should not call to you to the point of distraction. However, if the metabolism is not functioning normally and appetite receptors are not firing properly, food—especially high-sugar, high-fat, or high-calorie foods—may relentlessly beckon to you. While someone with normal appetite receptor function may pick up a handful of potato chips and move on, someone with a malfunctioning feedback loop will probably be distracted by the chips and will have to wage an internal battle in order to ignore the urge to eat all of them.

When is Enough Enough?

I refer to satisfaction as coming from two places: the brain and the stomach. Frequently, people with a metabolic problem might stop eating only because everyone around them has stopped or because their stomach feels overly full. They don't stop eating because their brain senses they have had enough to eat and they feel satisfied. Because of this, the eating experience of people with metabolic issues often feels urgent, a feeling that can lead to faster eating and greater food intake. This happens because brain receptors (MC3Rs) aren't registering the food intake and, therefore, fail to signal that the meal is over.

Another common symptom of a malfunctioning metabolism is feeling the need to think about what was eaten throughout the day before deciding what to eat next. Conversely, people with a normally functioning metabolic pathway never feel a need to think about what they have previously eaten. They eat what and how much they want or need each time they are hungry. Then they move on, never looking back. Their brain senses that it's time to stop eating, and their stomach feels satisfied and comfortable. This is why people with normally functioning metabolisms end their meals. It's a simple concept, but one that is foreign to many people who struggle with a malfunctioning metabolism and excess body weight.

Elizabeth had a lifelong struggle with her weight, which eventually led her to undergo gastric bypass surgery years ago. Although she initially experienced considerable weight loss after her surgery, her weight later steadily—and uncontrollably—increased. Out of desperation, Elizabeth asked her surgeon if a band could be put around her tiny remaining stomach pouch. When she found this was not possible, she felt completely hopeless. After enrolling in a medically supervised diet program with little success, she came to see me as a last resort.

When I tested Elizabeth, I found that her metabolic pathway was not working correctly and that her blood sugar was plummeting to very low levels immediately after she ate. After implementing medical treatment to address these underlying metabolic problems, her body weight decreased and her appetite normalized—without dieting.

"I used to be a secret junk and sugar eater," Elizabeth shared. "Now, I'm really not. It's not a conscious decision or that I'm trying to reform. I just don't want to drag a pie home anymore. I can just get a piece of pie if I want to. No one is saying I can't. There are no more rules for the first time in my life."

Elizabeth's observations highlight the impact of a faulty metabolic feedback loop on appetite and body weight. When the loop is realigned and the metabolic signals make their way successfully to the end of the central metabolic pathway, appetite and body weight respond automatically. If Elizabeth's eating behaviors and weight struggles of the past were behavioral rather than medical, how could a lifelong problem have changed so dramatically in a matter of weeks, solely through medical treatment?

Biology vs. Behavior

Scientists have found that cues for eating and moving are significantly affected by biological factors arising from the peripheral and central metabolic pathways. While not all of my patients with weight issues have problems with eating cues, the vast majority has a heightened appetite response, impaired satisfaction after meals, and frequent preoccupation with food. It is very important to note, however, that this is a *biological* problem caused by glitches in the metabolic feedback loop, not a *behavioral* problem.

My patients often tell me they can't have tempting food in their house or they'll eat it.

"I'm a smart person!" Helen complained. "I'm running a company. So why can't I be in charge of this? It's the one area of my life where I don't understand why I can't achieve my goals. I'm competent in every other area of my life."

"I never feel satisfied unless I eat four pounds of pasta," Christine admitted.

"An hour after finishing a large meal," Dan told me, "I'm craving Mexican food—I'm starving."

Although these responses are symptoms of underlying biological issues, people often blame them on lack of control and refer to indulging such cravings as binge eating, stress eating, emotional eating, or boredom eating. After treating hundreds of patients with appetite issues, however, it has become clear to me that these symptoms are actually caused by short circuits affecting a portion (or portions) of the metabolic pathway. The appetite receptors are not receiving the message that the body is adequately fueled, and therefore they are not allowing the appetite to calm down.

Once appetite cues are unbalanced, is there any hope of regaining normal innate eating habits? In my experience, the answer is "YES." Remarkably, with treatment targeted at improving the signaling throughout the metabolic pathway, symptoms can dissipate within days. Many of my patients report that for the first time in decades— or even for the first time ever—they actually experience "what it feels like to be normal" in terms of hunger, food interest, and satisfaction.

Like Elizabeth, patients who have regained metabolic balance report that food used to call out to them. "If I was at a bakery and saw some delicious-looking cake, I might buy the entire cake," one patient said. "But now I walk past the bakery and I'm not as interested. I might buy one piece of cake and feel free to enjoy it at a normal pace without feeling desperate or guilty, or without craving more." Other patients have said that even when they're enjoying their favorite meal and there is food left on their plate, they can now feel completely satisfied and naturally stop eating.

Indeed, most patients tell me that having normal appetite regulation—what people with normal metabolic function take for granted—is "an incredibly freeing experience."

Food Indecision

Although it's less common, metabolic impairment can also cause decreased appetite or an absence of appetite. Patients with this kind of metabolic issue tend to struggle with making food choices, either having trouble deciding between foods or feeling that nothing looks good. People whose metabolic pathway is working properly, in contrast, usually know what they want and can make a decision fairly quickly.

People with impaired metabolic function experience a great deal of indecision, often opening cabinets or standing in front of the refrigerator door, eating this or that or this *and* that, in an effort to satisfy their appetite. Some cope with their indecision by sticking to a fixed eating schedule, thereby avoiding the uncertainty of not knowing what to eat or feeling like they are not in control of what they eat.

I have observed that it is less common to experience an unusually decreased or absent appetite than it is to experience an overly increased appetite—but both issues are equally indicative of metabolic malfunction.

STEP 2: DIGESTION

Although we often associate *digestion* with the stomach, the digestive process actually begins in the mouth, where enzymes in the saliva begin breaking food down into components the body can absorb. When we chew, the body activates additional enzymes further down the gastrointestinal (GI) tract that help prepare the body to absorb the incoming nutrients, ready the pancreas for insulin production, and activate hormones in the gut that tell the brain we are eating, which is what makes us feel satiated.

The food then travels down the esophagus and into the stomach. Here, the *stretch receptors*, which are part of the nervous system, sense when the stomach is full. Meanwhile, a variety of hormones and enzymes coordinate the digestive process, helping the stomach break down the food, assisting absorption, and communicating to the rest of the body that we are eating.

Eventually, acids and enzymes in the stomach transform the food into liquid, making it easier for the body to absorb nutrients. The liquefied food then enters the small intestine—a narrow, 20-plus-foot-long tube that snakes between the stomach and large intestine—and the small intestine finishes digesting the food, breaking the macronutrients down into their smallest components: glucose and other sugars, amino acids, fatty acids, and micronutrients (vitamins and minerals).

People often complain that they feel bloated after eating. This happens when hormonal malfunctions cause the stomach to empty at irregular rates. Incretins (the hormones in the lower GI tract that we discussed in Chapter 3) regulate the pace at which the stomach empties, but when there are deficiencies of these hormones, our brain doesn't sense satiety, and the stomach can empty into the small intestine too rapidly. Because we don't feel full, we may increase the pace and quantity of our food intake, causing the stomach to become overly distended. Without normally functioning satiety cues, we begin to rely on this bloated feeling to know we've had enough to eat. In contrast, for a person with normal metabolic function, satiety cues are sensed in the brain first, followed by the stomach.

STEP 3: ABSORPTION

Tiny "fingers," or *villi*, that line the walls of the small intestine transport sugars, amino acids, fatty acids, vitamins, and minerals out of the intestine and into the bloodstream, which carries the nutrients throughout the body for utilization. When the metabolism is operating normally, the pace of nutrient absorption is perfectly matched to pancreas insulin production by hormones from the brain and GI tract, ensuring optimal nutrient processing and utilization. When the metabolism is mal-functioning, however, these hormones may be non-operational or deficient. This can make the pace of nutrient absorption irregular or too rapid, causing a mismatch of glucose with insulin and creating a suboptimal environment for nutrient processing and utilization.

STEP 4: UTILIZATION

When the body is well-tuned and feels secure that it has enough food and body mass, it will distribute absorbed nutrients based on the needs of its various parts and their functions.

A healthy metabolism paces itself, speeding up or slowing down fuel utilization based on the energy demands the body places upon it. This helps to explain why some people maintain a normal weight for their entire life—they have a healthy metabolism that manages their weight for them, keeping them in a normal range.

Metabolic Rates

Metabolic rate refers to the number of calories the body burns per minute to complete tasks at hand. The body's metabolic rate is continually set and adjusted by the metabolic feedback loop based on the brain and body's perception of body weight, food availability, and what activities are being performed.

The ability to measure metabolism by what is called *indirect calorimetry* was discovered in 1780. By the 1940s, scientists studying metabolism and obesity were routinely measuring metabolic response to various diets. Today's equipment is streamlined, comfortable for the patient, and much easier to use than the equipment used seventy years ago, but the concept behind it is the same: metabolism rates are determined by measuring the body's "exhaust" in a patient's exhaled breath.

Basal Metabolism

The majority of the calories we consume are burned while our body is running at its *basal metabolic rate* (BMR), the background burn rate at which it operates while we're sleeping. You would be surprised how much energy we expend lying flat on our back. Keeping the brain running, heart beating, blood flowing, lungs breathing, liver and kidneys functioning, and bowels moving—maintaining all the activities essential to life—requires a tremendous number of calories, and the body saves its heavy lifting for the night shift, when few other energy demands exist. For example, we grow and repair injured body parts while we're sleeping—whether it's tendons, ligaments, bones, organs, or skin. This is one reason why it's vital that we not skimp on sleep: it's critical for completing the metabolic processes of regeneration.

Resting Metabolism & Daily Metabolism Rates

The rate at which the metabolism operates when it's resting is higher than our basal metabolic rate, because it has to accommodate the additional energy we expend while awake and alert.

The *daily metabolic rate* differs from the *resting metabolic rate* because it includes the additional energy we expend when we're involved in our daily activities—showering, eating, moving around, caring for our children, driving to work, and so on.

Resting Metabolism: Fed State

The four hours or so that it takes to eat and digest a meal make up what we call the body's *fed metabolic state*. During this time, nutrients flow out of food and into the bloodstream, then the body divides the fuel up to either expend immediately or store for later. In its fed state, the body processes and burns what is immediately on hand rather than stored fat. While the body digests food, the metabolic rate raises about 10 percent above where it operates when we have not eaten. This effect of food upon the metabolic rate is referred to as its *thermogenic* effect.

Resting Metabolism: Fasting State

Beginning about four hours after we eat, after the main work of digestion is complete and the energy and nutrients from a meal have been apportioned, the resting metabolism re-enters its *fasting state*. Glucose no longer flows out of the food and into the bloodstream; instead, the liver's glycogen releases glucose into the bloodstream to balance blood sugar levels. The bloodstream then carries that glucose to the body cells, where it becomes the main source of energy between meals.

In its resting state, the metabolism normally burns equal amounts of carbohydrates (glucose) and fat, plus a very small amount of protein. If we don't eat enough carbohydrates, the body burns more protein because it can convert protein to carbohydrates. Since the brain must have glucose to operate normally, carbohydrates are essential for normal mood and brain function. The body cannot convert fats to carbohydrates, so if it needs more carbs, it takes proteins from the muscles and immune system to supply the needed energy. This results in muscle breakdown and reduced immune function.

Exercising Metabolism

Muscles usually can't absorb glucose from the blood-stream without help from the hormone insulin. However, during exercise only, the muscle cells—which are the most metabolically active cells in the body—have an additional way to access circulating glucose that doesn't require in-sulin. Muscle cells store carbohydrates as glycogen and fats as triglycerides in the form of liquid fuel droplets. The muscle cells can access immediate energy from these fuel droplets during exercise rather than having to wait for energy to arrive from elsewhere in the body. (By exercise I'm referring to any continuous motion that challenges the body, such as a jog, a swim, a bike ride, or even gar-dening or a brisk walk.) The muscle cells utilize whatever glycogen and triglycerides exist inside of them, and then, if necessary, they replenish themselves with glucose from the bloodstream to tank up energy stores for future use.

Regular, consistent exercisers and endurance athletes store more glycogen in their muscles than non-athletes. They need this extra fuel to meet the strenuous demands

JUST THE FACTS

Many misconceptions exist about exercise and burn-ing fat. The fat the body burns during exercise con-sists primarily of liquid droplets of fat stored in the muscles, not body fat from adipose tissue.

that they place on their body. About three hours of carbohydrate energy are stored in a trained athlete's muscles. In contrast, sedentary people store only enough energy in their muscles to react to immediate demands or emergencies. As you will learn in the next chapter, if someone has metabolic problems that include insulin resistance, their glycogen stores may be diminished due to the difficulty glucose has in getting into their muscle cells.

WORKING HARD, GETTING NOWHERE

Like appetite, the impetus to move—scientifically called *locomotive activity*—is also directly affected by the status of the metabolic pathway. For example, high levels of ghrelin, insulin resistance, and adiponectin malfunction have been found to affect the muscles' ability to store and access energy. In animal studies, forcibly increasing ghrelin levels in an animal's body has been shown to lead to a reduction of *ad lib locomotion*—meaning that the animal becomes sluggish and reduces its movement. When this problem is reversed in the laboratory and ghrelin levels return to normal, the animal immediately regains its movement and begins to exercise.[1]

---

1. I.D. Blum, Z. Patterson, R. Khazall, et al., "Reduced Anticipatory Locomotor Responses to Scheduled Meals in Ghrelin Receptor Deficient Mice," *Neuroscience* (December 8, 2009), doi: 10.1016/j.neuroscience.2009.08.009, PMCID: PMC2996828.

Humans are no different than laboratory mice in this regard: we directly respond to the body's perceptions of our energy balance. As you may recall from Chapter 3, the body's reaction to the perception of starvation can often be as strong as its reaction to actual starvation. Reduction in movement is part of the body's attempt to conserve energy and store fat for protection.

Over time, people with hormonal imbalances can feel increasingly tired, hungry, and eventually exhausted. Exercise, in particular, can become increasingly difficult, even uncomfortable. Not surprisingly, this can cause some people to become inactive. However, in spite of these serious challenges, many of my patients who struggle with weight issues are extremely athletic.

Meg has been an avid cyclist her entire life and commutes to work by bike several times a week—but in spite of her athleticism, she struggles with obesity, insulin resistance, and other metabolic issues. "I ride my bike all year round," she said. "I know I'm stronger and more fit than many of the cyclists I see on the road, but they are always passing me, especially on the hills. It's really frustrating and demoralizing. I'm a serious athlete, but I don't look or perform like one in spite of all my efforts."

Meg is in good company. In general, many of my patients are exercising far more and being more careful about their food intake than normal-weight people. I see some patients who have the fitness level of a competitive endurance athlete, but their performance doesn't even come close to reflecting their level of fitness. Due to the excess weight they are carrying, they expend a significant portion of their energy merely moving their body forward—which means that they are likely to be slower than their normal-weight competitors, regardless of their fitness level.

Thus many people become sedentary not because they don't want to exercise or because they're inherently lazy, but because exercise is much harder for them than it is for people with a normal metabolism. When metabolic hormones are balanced, people increase their locomotion; when their metabolism is blocked by hormonal imbalances, they decrease locomotion. The desire to be inactive is a biological and hormonal response, not simply a lifestyle choice.

A normally functioning metabolism can rev up or down as the situation warrants. For example, resting metabolic rate increases after exercise to help the body perform additional tasks, such as strengthening tissues and repairing micro-tears, in a process called *afterburn*. During afterburn, the resting metabolism increases slightly for a time period that can range from minutes to days, depending on the type of workout the person has engaged in. With an impaired metabolism, afterburn may not take place, which can lead to the metabolism rate actually decreasing in the hours after exercise in an attempt to compensate for a falsely perceived energy deficiency.

While many people with metabolism problems are avid athletes and feel great when they exercise, it makes sense that some people with metabolic problems complain of being tired after exercise and not experiencing the "exercise high" that many other people describe.

"I feel tired after exercise. I feel like I'm struggling through it," some of my patients complain. Others tell me, "I exercise first thing in the morning to get it out of the way because I hate it" or "People say exercise is refreshing, but I never feel invigorated afterward."

A HEALTHY METABOLISM:
FREE TO BURN FUEL

When the metabolism functions optimally, it stabilizes and balances the amount of energy we consume with the amount of energy we expend. We feel steady energy throughout the day. When we try to do more, our bodies provide us with more energy. Our weight consistently remains in a normal range without effort. Our brain and body maintain this balance by making often-imperceptible upward or downward adjustments that speed and slow our metabolism.

One way to think of healthy metabolic function is to compare it to driving a car. For example, say you want to drive a consistent 65 miles per hour. To stay at 65 you have to make adjustments: when you climb a hill or encounter a headwind, you press harder on the gas pedal so the car won't slow down; on the downslope, you let up on the gas or tap the brakes to slow down. Gas tank on "E"? Time to refuel.

A metabolism that operates normally is free to burn fuel at whatever rate the body requires. So when people with a healthy metabolism eat more than usual at a party or while they're on vacation, their body automatically speeds up and burns the extra fuel. If they work late and delay dinner for several hours or even skip a meal, their body taps the brakes, causing the metabolism to slow down to preserve energy until the next meal. People without weight issues don't try to control their weight by eating less or exercising more. They don't have to—their metabolism automatically balances how much energy they consume with how much they expend.

TAKING CRUISE CONTROL FOR GRANTED

Even though science tells us a healthy metabolism auto-matically balances fuel consumption, the story set forth in popular culture is that this balancing act requires will-power and control. According to this theory, people who don't have a weight problem or whose weight remains stable achieve this through control and willpower—by eating carefully and exercising regularly. They do everything right, which means that everyone else must be doing things wrong. When we stop to think, however, and we ignore these popular culture messages, we know this is absurd. Not only is this explanation unscientific, it's illogical.

Everyone knows somebody who eats freely or who doesn't exercise at all yet doesn't have a weight problem. Everyone also knows somebody who is careful about eating and exercise yet battles with weight—it might even be you. It's very hard to believe that a person who has never struggled with weight eats the exact same number of calories and burns that exact same number of calories every single day, day in and day out, year after year. That's what would have to happen if the conventional wisdom about the relationship between diets, exercise, and weight was hard science.

People whose metabolisms function normally often don't know a different way of being, thus they may take their normal appetite and their body's weight-balancing for granted. They may even wrongly believe that their diet and exercise choices are what allow their weight to remain stable. I've heard normal-weight people say more than once that if overweight people would just do everything they did, they would not have a weight problem.

WEIGHT-PRONE OR WEIGHT-RESISTANT: A MATTER OF CHANCE

Science shows us that normal-weight people are far less responsible for their weight than they may believe.

If normal-weight people are not as responsible for their weight as we have been led to believe, then logic tells us overweight people may not be responsible for theirs, either. Scientific research amassed over the past one hundred years supports this perspective; so do the cases I've witnessed firsthand in the twenty-five years I've spent treating overweight patients in my clinical practice. Weight problems most frequently develop because the metabolism is experiencing an imbalance—not because a patient is doing something wrong.

CHAPTER 5

A History of Ideas

OVER THE YEARS, THERE have been many theories about what causes obesity and overweight conditions. Some were bizarre; others made a lot of sense. Some people thought it was overeating and lack of exercise; others thought it was depression and psychological problems. Treatments for overweight have included "starvation therapy" in the early 1900s (which carried a high mortality rate), as well as medically supervised diets and exercise, which have been administered since before the 1920s. In the 1950s, theories of depression being the root cause of weight problems led to a focus on behavioral therapy, which is still popular today. Up through the present time, the medical community—and society in general—have continued to focus on diets, exercise, and behavioral treatment as the answer to obesity and overweight.

Dr. Lulu Hunt Peters, who herself struggled with weight problems, was one of the first diet advocates. In her best-selling book *Diet & Health*, published in 1918, she referred to obese people as "fireless cookers" who were prone to store fat and therefore required strict caloric guidelines.

> . . . *Thin people have been proved to radiate fifty percent more heat per pound than fat people; in other words, fat people are regular fireless cookers! They hold the heat in, it cannot get out through the packing, and the food which is also contained therein goes merrily on with fiendish regularity, depositing itself as fat.*[1]

While Dr. Hunt Peters accredited her health and vitality to strict adherence to her own dieting advice, she lived to only 57 years of age before succumbing to pneumonia.

---

1. Lulu Hunt Peters, *Diet and Health with Key to the Calories*, (Chicago: The Reilly and Lee Co., 1918): Ch. 1.

AHEAD OF THEIR TIME

Many scientific journal articles from the 1920s and '30s reveal that physicians pondered obesity in a much more analytical way than many physicians do today. One of my favorite historical accounts of the science of obesity and metabolism is from Dr. Hans Lisser's 1924 publication "The Frequency of Endogenous Endocrine Obesity and its Treatment by Glandular Therapy."[2]

Lisser's presentation to the 53rd Annual Session of the California Medical Board and the comments in response to it show the insight that physicians of his day had in spite of their limited resources. In his presentation, Dr. Lisser explained why diet and exercise could not be considered a cure:

> *Radical diet restriction often reduces weight, but cannot be termed a "cure" because it fails to correct the fundamental cause of such incretory obesity . . . The chemistry of obesity is still quite obscure . . . Several glands exert a powerful influence on the shape and bulk of the human body.*

---

2. H. Lisser, "The Frequency of Endogenous Endocrine Obesity and Its Treatment By Glandular Therapy," *Western Journal of Medicine* (October 1924), 22(10): 509–514.

Lisser pointed out that some people are clearly weight-prone, and some are clearly weight-resistant.

Most of us are acquainted with people who eat lightly and are very active, but who nevertheless accumulate fatty tissue. Likewise, we are aware that many persons eat heartily, are not especially athletic, and yet remain thin.

Based on his understanding of the science of his day and his observations of his own patients, Lisser concluded that diet and exercise could not "cure" the underlying cause of a weight problem, and he was eager to address the root cause rather than apply a treatment that had little chance of succeeding in the long term.

. . . Normal food intake and normal exercise will not avail with such individuals because an underlying factor is responsible which is not sufficiently recognized in diagnosis and not given proper consideration in planning treatment. This factor is an abnormal faulty metabolism, the control of which is to a large extent dominated by the glands of internal secretion.

As Lisser discusses below, even in 1924, the science—including standard endocrinology textbooks—clearly stated that hormonal issues underlie weight problems, and that excess weight is a symptom of those issues. Knowing that the theory that diets and exercise were not a cure was radical to some, Lisser carefully reminded the reader that that these were not his ideas—they were established science represented in a wide range of textbooks at the time.

It is obviously beyond the confines of this paper to describe in detail the various types of ductless gland disease in which obesity is a common and prominent symptom . . . Many excellent text-books are available, such as Falta, Cushing, Barker in Monographic Medicine, etc. There is nothing original in the observation that obesity is a striking symptom of incretory deficiencies.

Many of the authors referenced here by Lisser remain famous today, including Cushing, the endocrinologist who discovered Cushing's disease.

Lisser recognized that irregular appetite is a symptom of the underlying glitches in the metabolic feedback loop. His insight in this area stemmed from research being done at the time that examined what happened in rodents when parts of the brain were cut off from communication with other parts. He didn't know that the reason for the appetite changes was specifically due to impairment of MC3R activity—however, he did realize that hormones from the pituitary gland must have a role in appetite regulation, metabolic rate, and weight control.

A large appetite and a craving for sweets and starches may characterize a glutton, but it is to be remembered that this craving may itself be pathological, and depend on hypopituitarism. The hunger, thirst, and high sugar tolerance of these patients is well known. A mere restriction of food intake only scratches the surface, but neglects the underlying cause. Results would be temporary, because the patient rarely persists against an abnormal appetite difficult to control. Gland administration to supplement the patient's gland deficiency is a sound logical procedure.

In 1934, ten years after Lisser's influential paper was published, British doctor A.H. Douthwaite upheld the theory of appetite as a potential symptom rather than the cause of obesity:[3]

There is no evidence to prove that increased appetite is the primary cause of obesity. It is

---

3. A.H. Douthwaite, "The Treatment Of Obesity," *The British Medical Journal* (August 15, 1936), Vol. 2, No. 3945: 844.

conceivable that another factor, "the undeter-
minable tendency to obesity," may in itself be
responsible for the increased appetite.

Here, Dr. Douthwaite contemplates the possibilities of a neuroendocrine cause of the problem:

In certain instances, disease of the central ner-
vous system or dysfunction of the endocrine
glands so affects the metabolism of the body as
to favor and accelerate the generalized or local-
ized deposition of fat.

While the specific details have been better clarified in more recent years, Drs. Lisser, Douthwaite, and their colleagues were certainly on the right track in their efforts to outline the function of the central and peripheral metabolic pathways; in fact, their theories are still extremely current in terms of the modern scientific view of obesity's causes and potential treatments.

THE UNTOLD STORY

Dr. Lisser's theories about obesity were well received by many of the endocrinology greats of the 1920s and '30s, but the general viewpoint was still that gluttony was the cause of weight problems. It seemed logical that a person who was gaining weight was doing so because they were eating too much. Experts did not likely understand the weight defense system in the early 1900s, which is when some of them began encouraging diets. It was not until the 1940s and later that scientists and doctors began to realize that every type of diet they devised had a side effect: slowing of the metabolic rate.

Fortunately, scientists have made great strides in mapping out the neuroendocrine control of the metabolism, body weight, and appetite since the early 1900s. Even in 1924, scientists were already beginning to sharply challenge the "calories in, calories out" explanation of weight gain, and scientists today know that this theory is an oversimplification. We can now identify and measure many factors that not only trip the body's starvation defenses but also trigger a cascade of hormonal reactions, rendering "calories out" unpredictable and inaccurate. "Calories in, calories out" simply doesn't account for how the weight defense system impacts the rate at which the body burns energy.

Surprisingly, in spite of the impressive body of knowledge that now exists about these topics, we still cling to a nearly one-hundred-year-old theory about why we gain weight and how to address weight problems. This is especially puzzling because the "calories in, calories out" perspective and corresponding behavioral treatments have clearly been ineffective: Americans today are actually eating less but weighing more.[4]

In the article "Obesity: Overnutrition or disease of metabolism?", published in 1953 in the *American Journal of Digestive Diseases*,[5] A.W. Pennington describes his review of past studies showing that fat storage appears to be independent of energy intake:

> *Analysis of the results of studies of the energy exchange in obesity, in regard to their evidence for or against a passive dependence of the excessive energy stores on the balance between the inflow and the outflow of energy, indicates that these stores have a significant degree of independence of the energy balance.*
>
> *This appears to necessitate an explanation of obesity on the basis of some intrinsic metabolic defect.*

---

4. E.S. Ford, W.H. Dietz, "Trends in energy intake among adults in the United States: findings from NHANES," *American Journal of Clinical Nutrition* (February 20, 2013), doi: 10.3945/ajcn.112.052662.

5. A.W. Pennington, "Obesity: Overnutrition or disease of metabolism?," *American Journal of Digestive Diseases* (September 1953), Vol. 20, Issue 9: 268-274.

Pennington also noted that when normal-weight and overweight subjects dieted, they *both* experienced a reduction in their metabolic rate as a side effect.

The decline in energy expenditure which occurs when the obese go on low calorie diets appears to have the same significance as it has when people of normal weight are subjected to undernutrition.

In his conclusion, Pennington argues that, rather than create calorie restriction (go on a diet), the solution to obesity would be to target fat stores in the body.

A treatment of obesity, alternate to that of caloric restriction, takes into account the metabolic defect in obesity, aims at a primary decrease in the excessive energy stores, and allows for weight reduction without any decline in the energy expenditure and without any enforcement of caloric restriction.

Pennington was challenging the thinking of his time, but it seems he could not completely disconnect from the diet approach: he went on to experiment with liberal-calorie, low-carb diets, all of which effected only short-term success. In the process, he developed the theory that Atkins later popularized and the Paleo diet modernized. Essentially, many people today are following a diet that was first tried—without long-term success—sixty years ago.

Another article published in the *Journal of Clinical Endocrinology and Metabolism* in 1984,[6] also found that after a diet, a patient's metabolism slowed by an amount that was proportionate to the amount of weight lost—the equivalent of 450 calories daily for someone who loses fifty pounds by dieting. This article was published thirty years after Pennington had stated that the research of his time proved this same theory: the more weight was lost, the more the metabolism slowed. E. Jéquier wrote:

> *After weight loss, energy expenditure decreases by about 84 kJ/24 h (20 kcal/24 h) per kg of weight loss in all patients. The need to reset energy intake to a lower level than the previous maintenance food consumption represents a major difficulty in the treatment of obesity; failure to adjust energy intake to the new requirements contributes to the frequent relapse of body weight gain in the obese after completion of a period on a hypocaloric diet.*

---

6. E. Jéquier, "Energy expenditure in obesity," *Journal of Clinical Endocrinology & Metabolism* (November 1984): 563-580.

THE SAME OLD STORY

People often assume that as long as you exercise, your metabolism won't drop with dieting. But scientists have proven that this assumption is false. In 2012, for example, scientists performed a "biggest loser"-style weight-loss diet program and measured metabolic changes. Their results confirmed past studies: after thirty weeks of dieting and intense exercise to preserve muscle mass, subjects lost thirty percent of their body weight, but their metabolisms slowed by 500 calories per day.[7]

More recent studies have examined the hormonal mechanisms behind the slowing of metabolism. An article published in the *New England Journal of Medicine* in 2011, titled "Long-term persistence of hormonal adaptations to weight loss,"[8] described a study of fifty overweight and obese patients who participated in a ten-week, very low-calorie diet. Hormone levels were measured once before the diet and twice after the diet, once at ten weeks and once at sixty-two weeks. Researchers found that the diet left a lasting fingerprint on participants' levels of several hormones, including leptin and insulin, and put them in a protective mode (Diet Fog) that was likely to lead to weight regain.

7. D.L. Johannsen, N.D.Knuth, "Metabolic Slowing with Massive Weight Loss despite Preservation of Fat-Free Mass," *Journal of Clinical Endocrinology & Metabolism* (2012), 97(7): 2489-2496.

8. P. Sumithran, L.A. Prendergast , et al., "Long-term persistence of hormonal adaptations to weight loss," *New England Journal of Medicine* (October 27, 2011), 365(17), doi: 10.1056/NEJMoa1105816: 1597-1604.

One year after initial weight reduction, levels of the circulating mediators of appetite that encourage weight regain after diet-induced weight loss do not revert to the levels recorded before weight loss. Long-term strategies to counteract this change may be needed to prevent obesity relapse.

The researchers also found that patients had regained a significant amount of the weight they lost and had much higher hunger ratings.

Yet another recent study by the same researchers, published in *Clinical Science* in 2013,[9] examines the chemical changes during Diet Fog that occur as a result of dieting.

Diet-induced weight loss is accompanied by several physiological changes which encourage weight regain, including alterations in energy expenditure, substrate metabolism and hormone pathways involved in appetite regulation, many of which persist beyond the initial weight loss period.

---

9. P. Sumithran, J. Proietto, "The defense of body weight: a physiological basis for weight regain after weight loss," *Clinical Science* (February 2013), 124(4), doi: 10.1042/CS20120223: 231-241.

CENTURIES OF DISCOVERY:

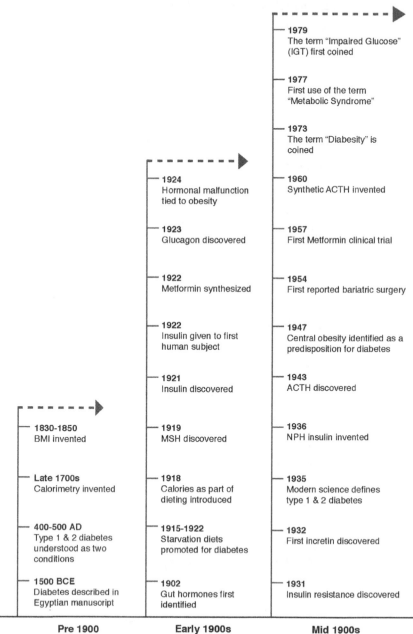

1979
The term "Impaired Glucose" (IGT) first coined

1977
First use of the term "Metabolic Syndrome"

1973
The term "Diabesity" is coined

1924
Hormonal malfunction tied to obesity

1960
Synthetic ACTH invented

1923
Glucagon discovered

1957
First Metformin clinical trial

1922
Metformin synthesized

1954
First reported bariatric surgery

1922
Insulin given to first human subject

1947
Central obesity identified as a predisposition for diabetes

1921
Insulin discovered

1943
ACTH discovered

1830-1850
BMI invented

1919
MSH discovered

1936
NPH insulin invented

Late 1700s
Calorimetry invented

1918
Calories as part of dieting introduced

1935
Modern science defines type 1 & 2 diabetes

400-500 AD
Type 1 & 2 diabetes understood as two conditions

1915-1922
Starvation diets promoted for diabetes

1932
First incretin discovered

1500 BCE
Diabetes described in Egyptian manusoript

1902
Gut hormones first identified

1931
Insulin resistance discovered

Pre 1900   **Early 1900s**   **Mid 1900s**

DIETING, HORMONES, DISEASES & TREATMENTS

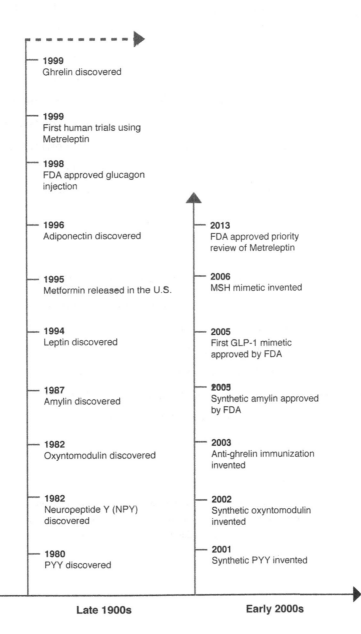

1999
Ghrelin discovered

1999
First human trials using
Metreleptin

1998
FDA approved glucagon
injection

1996
Adiponectin discovered

1995
Metformin released in the U.S.

1994
Leptin discovered

1987
Amylin discovered

1982
Oxyntomodulin discovered

1982
Neuropeptide Y (NPY)
discovered

1980
PYY discovered

2013
FDA approved priority
review of Metreleptin

2006
MSH mimetic invented

2005
First GLP-1 mimetic
approved by FDA

2005
Synthetic amylin approved
by FDA

2003
Anti-ghrelin immunization
invented

2002
Synthetic oxyntomodulin
invented

2001
Synthetic PYY invented

Late 1900s   **Early 2000s**

Over the decades, researchers have proven time and time again that dieting is a short-term strategy that triggers the body's weight defenses. The body can detect deprivation—you can't trick it into losing weight long-term by reducing your calorie intake—so dieting has little chance of solving weight problems in the long run.

Even before Pennington's time, hundreds of studies showed the same results. Information about diets not working in the long term and about diets slowing the metabolism is now included as established fact in every textbook on obesity or metabolism. So why hasn't public opinion changed?

CHALLENGING OUR ASSUMPTIONS

Recent research has expanded the scientific investigation of weight problems to associations other than dieting and exercise. For example, a study examining snacking in teens shows that teens who snacked were not at increased risk of obesity, and in fact some studies show that teens who snack are at a lower risk for obesity, even when their snacks are fast food-based.[10]

---

10. N. Larson, et al., "A review of snacking patterns among children and adolescents: what are the implications of snacking for weight status," *Child Obesity Journal* (April 2013), 9(2) doi: 10.1089/chi.2012.0108: 104-115.

One study examined the association between sleep and teens with a propensity for overweight: it found that teens who slept more than 7.5 hours per night showed a lower risk for obesity.[11] Another study revealed that nearly 7,000 kids who participated in an intensive physical activity program in school exhibited no association between their activity and their body weight or body fat levels.[12] Still other studies have shown that "food deserts"— places where there is a lack of fresh food and increased availability of fast food—are actually not associated with an increased risk of overweight and obesity.[13]

In the face of the repeated long-term failures of diets, many researchers are still talking about trying to figure out how to trick the body into not sensing deprivation during deprivation diets. I, however, strongly believe— based on almost one hundred years of research, as well as the success I've had with my patients—that the better

11. J.A. Mitchell, D. Rodriguez, et al., "Sleep Duration and Adolescent Obesity," *Pediatrics* (April 8, 2013), doi: 10.1542/peds: 2012-2368.

12. J. Deardorff, "Measuring body fat may weigh on students' self-image," *Chicago Tribune,* June 9, 2013.

13. D. Viola, P.S. Arno, A.R. Maroko, et al., "Overweight and obesity: Can we reconcile evidence about supermarkets and fast food retailers for public health policy?," *Journal of Public Health Policy* (May 30, 2013), doi: 10.1057/jphp.2013.19.

approach is to apply the science of metabolism and avoid diets altogether. Why diet or try to trick our bodies when we can potentially detect and correct the true underlying causes of overweight and obesity, rendering those other measures unnecessary?

CHAPTER 6

Metabolic Storm and Diet Fog: A Veritable Firewall

WEIGHT PROBLEMS OCCUR for many reasons, but most have genetic roots—in fact, scientists believe that up to .70 percent of obesity is genetically based. A combination of genetic and environmental factors creates glitches in the metabolic feedback loop, causing the body and brain to inaccurately perceive starvation. Potential triggers of this malfunction include:

- puberty hormones
- medications (certain antidepressants or psychotropic medications, birth control,

steroids like prednisone and cortisone
shots, most sleeping medications, and
certain cholesterol and blood pressure
medications)

- environmental toxins (found in cosmet-
ics, plastics, fragrances, pollution, pesti-
cides, etc.)
- sleep deprivation or sleep apnea
- dieting or under-fueled exercise

METABOLIC STORM

When glitches in our metabolic feedback loop cause the
body to perceive that we are starving, it acts defensively,
simultaneously lowering our metabolic rate and compel-
ling us to consume more fuel. If we ignore this drive to
eat, our body simply slows our metabolism even further
in an attempt to meet its protective goal of defending or
increasing its fat mass. I refer to the powerful malfunctions of the metabolic feedback loop that promote and
protect excess body weight as the Metabolic Storm.

There are numerous common warning signs of an
underlying hormonal imbalance, and they differ among
people—in fact, a person can experience different warning signs at different times throughout their life. These
include:

- constant hunger
- not feeling satisfied after eating
- frequent and sudden feelings of an overly full stomach
- a preoccupation with food
- indecision about whether to eat and what to eat
- cravings for sweets or high-fat foods
- low energy
- reproductive system issues in both men and women (irregular periods, low testosterone, and infertility, precocious puberty in girls, slowing of height increase in adolescents)

THESE GLITCHES ARE BITCHES

Short circuits in the metabolic feedback loop activate a series of defenses that adjust the behavior of not just one hormone or body system, but *several* of them—and all at once. These adjustments form a veritable firewall against body fat loss and, ultimately, starvation. The brain and body may have activated the weight defense system based on an inaccurate perception of the situation, but their goal is no different than it would be were they experiencing actual starvation: to defend body mass by causing metabolic slowdown and weight gain.

There are numerous hormonal glitches that can cause disproportionate weight gain or weight-loss resistance, including insulin resistance, adiponectin deficiency, low leptin, leptin resistance, incretin deficiency, amylin malfunction, and ghrelin excess. As you will discover, all of these malfunctions can result in elevated blood sugar, insulin imbalance, slowing metabolism, weight gain, and appetite deregulation. We'll begin with insulin resistance.

Insulin Resistance

You may remember that insulin helps bring glucose and proteins into the body tissues so they can utilize it for energy. By removing glucose from the blood and carrying it into the tissues, insulin helps keep blood glucose from getting too high. Insulin also reassures the brain that we are nourished. One of the many ways in which the body accumulates fat is through a medical problem called *insulin resistance*.

Insulin resistance is characterized by a lack of response by the muscle tissue and the brain to the effects of insulin. This resistance makes it more difficult for glucose to enter the cells—potentially leading to an increase in circulating blood glucose and to signals telling the body to store rather than burn fat. This is a very common problem among overweight and obese people struggling with weight gain. Luckily, insulin resistance is reversible—but if left untreated, the pancreas's insulin-producing cells can eventually fatigue, increasing the risk of glucose buildup in the blood. At this point, insulin resistance progresses to pre-diabetes and then type 2 diabetes, which is why I often call insulin resistance "pre-pre-diabetes."

Insulin resistance can exist as part of *metabolic syndrome*, the diagnosis criteria being a minimum of three of the following features:

- elevated glucose or insulin levels
- cholesterol abnormalities (elevated triglycerides, elevated LDL particles, and/or low HDL)
- elevated blood pressure
- increased abdominal circumference

In women, insulin resistance can also be associated with a condition called *polycystic ovarian syndrome* (PCOS). PCOS is characterized by irregular menses, increased facial hair growth, acne, and infertility. There are lab tests that can detect PCOS, and a pelvic ultrasound can sometimes reveal numerous tiny ovarian cysts.

In men, insulin resistance can contribute to low testosterone and sometimes excess estrogen. Symptoms of these hormonal imbalances in men include increased

belly fat, increased breast tissue, low energy, poor con-
centration, and low sex drive.

Scientists have found that insulin resistance may
develop as a result of deeper underlying malfunctions.
One of these potential triggers can be an adiponectin
deficiency. As you may recall, adiponectin is an insulin
sensitizer, so when it declines, muscle insulin sensitivity
also can decline, causing insulin resistance. For other patients, inappropriately high insulin spikes after meals can
cause dramatic drops in blood sugar. When this happens
repeatedly, the body may eventually become resistant to
the excessive circulating insulin.

A common symptom of insulin resistance can be sugar
cravings, because the muscles feel starved of glucose. A fairly
frequent physical sign of the disorder is *acanthosis nigricans*,
a condition characterized by a darkening and thickening of
skin in the folds of the body and on the knuckles. Stretch
marks can also occur in people suffering from insulin
resistance, particularly darker-skinned people.

Research has shown that weight gain is often a symptom—not a cause—of insulin resistance. In insulin resistance, high insulin turns the body's fat burning switch
off and the fat storing switch on. As belly fat increases,
however, it contributes to the problem by releasing specialized hormones that exacerbate insulin resistance and
promote even more fat gain. This vicious cycle is a good

example of how metabolic hormones communicate with and support each other in a sometimes misguided attempt to ensure the body's survival.

As excess insulin makes blood vessels stiffer and thicker, the passageway through them narrows, a condition called *hypertrophy*. Hypertrophy increases blood pressure and can cause small blood vessels to close up, leading to heart attack or stroke.

People with a family history of diabetes, with a personal history of insulin resistance, pre-diabetes or gestational diabetes, or who were born to a mother who had gestational diabetes, are at a higher risk of developing diabetes. However, not everyone with insulin resistance is destined to develop diabetes—especially if they take steps to treat their condition.

Break A World Record, Win Olympic Medals— But "Put the Waffle Down, Margaret!"

Margaret[1] dreamed of becoming an Olympic swimmer from a young age—and she eventually reached that goal, participating in two Olympic Games. In 2008, while competing in her second Olympic Games in Beijing, Margaret won two silver medals and one bronze medal.

---

1. Margaret Hoelzer gave permission to use her real name in this book.

At one point in her career she even held a world record in the 200-meter backstroke.

As early as age eleven, however, and throughout her swimming career, no matter how hard Margaret trained, she struggled with her weight. "Even being as fit as I was, my coaches were never happy with my weight," she recalled.

With trainers pushing her to improve her body composition, Margaret restricted the types of foods she ate and cut both her calorie and her carb intake for years. She always felt tired, and she noticed that it took her longer to recover from workouts than it did her teammates. Even at the top of her game—even while holding a world record—her coaches basically told her to "put the waffle down." She was the fastest swimmer in the world in her signature event, the 200-meter backstroke, and yet she still wasn't good enough.

"I knew that my body was different when I compared myself to my college roommates. I watched how they ate. I ate no differently than they did, but I was bigger. It was more difficult for my weight to balance in a range normally attributed to highly competitive swimmers," Margaret said. The fact that she didn't "fit the profile" physically was very distressing to her, as her coaches continually focused on cutting back her food and her rest.

Finally, Margaret decided that she had had enough. Tired of feeling run down and hungry, she retired. As soon as she stopped her heavy Olympic-level training, however, Margaret gained weight rapidly. That's when she came to see me.

Like most patients struggling with weight, I discovered that Margaret had an underlying medical problem: insulin resistance. This condition, in addition to the strict diet and intense exercise regimen she had adhered to for many years, was causing her body to fiercely defend her weight. Although even Olympic athletes are rarely screened for them, the types of problems Margaret was experiencing are actually very common.

Like many other patients who struggle with their weight, Margaret burst into tears when I explained that her weight problems weren't her fault. "My entire life I'd been told that it was something I was doing wrong," she cried.

Not true. And imagine what such an accomplished champion could have achieved if she had not been battling a metabolic problem the entire time she was competing, and hadn't been starved and tired to boot.

The fact that insulin resistance causes the body to store fat is one of the most important reasons we have far less control over our weight than popular culture purports. People with insulin resistance can eat the same foods in the same quantities as people without the condition, but their body stores more fat in response, making it virtually impossible for them to lose weight.

Adiponectin Deficiency

In a normally functioning metabolism, fat emits adiponectin to inform the rest of the body about how much fat it's carrying. Adiponectin helps lean mass become more sensitive to insulin, allowing glucose to enter the tissue cells more easily. Adiponectin also increases metabolic rate and reduces inflammation throughout the body and within blood vessels.

But sometimes adiponectin levels drop. Scientists have observed that this malfunction can occur suddenly, as though something pulled a "trigger" metabolically. Many medications and environmental toxins common to our daily life have been implicated as possible culprits. Researchers believe that people with a genetic predisposition for diabetes are more vulnerable to "obesogens," which are environmental chemicals that disrupt the endocrine system, altering adiponectin and other metabolic hormone levels.

Obesogens include common household toxins like bisphenol A (BPA), phthalates, and other chemicals.

A recent study showed that teen girls who tested as having the highest BPA levels also had the highest BMIs.[2] Similar to many earlier studies, this showed a direct correlation between environmental toxins and metabolic

---

2. C. Petrochko, "BPA Level Tied to Higher Weight in Girls," *MedPage Today* (June 12, 2013).

issues. Metabolic disruption has also been traced to the womb, so there is no way to know if a suppression of adiponectin has occurred prenatally.

Some of my patients can identify a specific time in their life when their body weight became difficult to control, and it's often tied to when they started taking a particular medication. Most sleep medications—antianxiety, antipsychotic, and antidepressant medications; certain cholesterol and blood pressure medications; certain pain medications; prednisone and cortisone shots; and some forms of birth control or progesterone—can cause metabolic disruptions, including adiponectin suppression.

In addition to promoting insulin resistance, an adiponectin deficiency can also reduce the body's metabolic burn rate, both at rest and during exercise. In fact, many studies have shown that overweight children and adults frequently burn less fuel when they're resting and exercising than do normal-weight people.

Low Leptin

Fat cells emit leptin to inform the brain and body of body mass and fat status. With normal metabolic function, leptin levels represent body mass accurately, and we feel satisfied after eating. The body burns glucose normally and doesn't store excess fat. Normal body weight is maintained automatically with no added effort. But dieting (which is the most common cause of leptin suppression), under-fueled exercise, or low-blood-sugar reactions can suppress leptin levels disproportionate to the amount of body mass. In dieting, for example, fat begins to emit abnormally low amounts of leptin; in essence, the fat mass is hiding by emitting less leptin, blinding the brain from seeing the fat stores and making it believe the body weighs much less than it actually does.

This state, also called *hypoleptinemia* or *acquired leptin insufficiency*, is triggered by and accentuates the body's weight defense response. The brain and body shift into energy-conservation mode, storing fat. This is what is happening during the diet plateau and subsequent re-gain period. Once leptin drops very low, the metabolism slows and hunger becomes a biological response. Weight gain, then, is not the result of going off a diet; biology actually stops the weight loss and starts the weight gain *before* a diet ends. From the brain and body's distorted perspective, the body is not merely undernourished—it no longer carries enough fat tissue to ensure survival.

Leptin levels can drop unnaturally low in as little as seventy-two hours after a person starts dieting. These hor-monal changes that trigger the weight-defense system in response to restrictive eating—what I refer to as Diet Fog—are the underlying cause of the short-lived success of diets.

Scientists have repeatedly found that after a twelve-week diet and exercise program, leptin levels often remain suppressed for a minimum of one to two years. Leptin can also drop due to inadequate sleep. Cutting back on food intake to squeeze into a wedding dress, participating in a "detox," or trying to make weight for a sports event can push the body beyond its tipping point and into self-preservation mode.

Leptin Resistance

Leptin resistance causes the brain and body to wrongly believe that the body isn't carrying sufficient fat for survival. This triggers the body's weight defense system—shutting down metabolism, increasing the appetite, reducing satiety, and causing the body to conserve energy and store more fat.

In my practice, I often see leptin resistance in patients following a period of dieting. Leptin levels can drop dramatically during a diet—disproportionate to the amount of weight lost. After dropping, it may eventually sharply rebound to an abnormally high level, or to a normal level, but with impaired signaling in the brain. Increased ghrelin or decreased amylin (both known side effects of dieting) can be the cause of this impaired signaling—ghrelin by blocking leptin's signals, and amylin by failing to help the brain see the leptin. Leptin resistance can also be aggravated by sleep apnea.

Some of the most important receptor sites that can become resistant to leptin signals reside in the brain, liver, and pancreas. These sites significantly impact weight, glucose, and insulin regulation. The metabolic pathway breaks down when the brain is resistant to leptin signals—the appetite receptors don't receive signals that the body has sufficient mass, and the metabolism slows, resulting in the symptoms I've described before: an increased urge to forage, constant hunger, and a lack of satiety after eating.

This metabolic backlash is characterized by an acceleration of weight regain to at least the point of the pre-diet weight, and frequently beyond it—and once this process is initiated, it's difficult to bring under control.

Incretin Deficiency

Another way the metabolism can fool the brain into thinking it's starving and it should preserve and store body fat is by turning down or turning off incretins like GLP-1. This *incretin malfunction* occurs in dieting, anorexia, pre-diabetes, and diabetes. Deficient incretin levels cause miscommunication in the metabolic feedback loop: the brain doesn't receive the signal confirming fuel has been consumed. When this occurs, people often continue to feel hungry and unsatisfied in spite of having had a normal-sized meal, and the metabolism slows.

With deficient GLP-1, in addition to the brain not

acknowledging consumed fuel, the stomach empties faster and the gut takes the brakes off the pace at which glucose and other nutrients pass into the bloodstream, causing blood glucose levels to elevate. As a result, the body stores more glucose than normal as fat.

Amylin Malfunction

People with metabolic problems can frequently be either *amylin resistant* or *amylin deficient*. Amylin is secreted from the pancreas with insulin, so when insulin output is high, amylin output is as well. When hormone levels become too high, receptors lose their sensitivity to amylin and become resistant to its effects. On the other hand, people who diet or have anorexia may instead experience *suppressed* insulin and amylin output, causing them to be *amylin deficient*. In either case, there are similar metabolic consequences.

Amylin's major functions are to make the brain see the leptin signal more clearly and to regulate the pace of stomach emptying, nutrient absorption, and glucagon secretion from the pancreas. Amylin signaling problems can cause: the brain to remain resistant to leptin even when leptin levels are normal; rapid stomach emptying that pours a flood of nutrients into the bloodstream, triggering excess insulin output from the pancreas; and rapid glucagon secretion after meals, triggering glucose dumping from the liver into the bloodstream.

Ghrelin Excess

Ghrelin is secreted by the stomach. In normal conditions, ghrelin increases during fasting and before meals. *Ghrelin excess* is usually triggered by dieting or anorexia, though sleep deprivation and sleep apnea can also contribute. With ghrelin excess, baseline ghrelin levels elevate above normal and do not decline after eating—which means that although the body has been fueled, ghrelin continues to signal to the brain that there is a need for food.

People often refer to ghrelin as the "hunger hormone," but my patients with high ghrelin levels don't necessarily report feeling excessively hungry. The primary symptom that patients report is persistent, steady, and sometimes rapid weight gain, and weight-loss resistance in spite of all their efforts. In combination with decreased leptin and amylin, increased ghrelin usually precipitates weight-regain backlash after a diet—and it can get "stuck" in an elevated position, contributing to long-term weight-loss resistance.

DIET FOG: ONE THING ON TOP OF ANOTHER

Once an underlying hormonal imbalance develops, whether in early childhood or not until adulthood, people often find themselves between a rock and a hard place. If they diet, they temporarily lose weight, but regardless of how much they shed, the weight always seems to eventually return.

When a person with metabolic pathway glitches goes on a diet, Diet Fog always sets in at some point, creating a secondary problem that amplifies the underlying Metabolic Storm. Symptoms of Diet Fog are:

- plateau in weight loss while on a diet
- weight gain while on a diet
- return of extreme hunger after a period of increased satisfaction that occurred with the diet
- fatigue
- intense fear of weight regain while on a diet

Once the body sees the diet as deprivation, a starvation response kicks into gear—the brain and body essentially dial 911, mobilizing resources in order to survive. Scientific research has shown that a person's metabolism can slow by *400 to 500 calories a day* within weeks of beginning to diet. This helps to explain why most dieters plateau and then eventually gain back the weight that they lost (and often even more than that)—500 calories is what many people cut out of their daily intake when they diet, so when their metabolism slows that much, they're barely breaking even.

Just as you might turn down your thermostat and unplug appliances to reduce your carbon footprint or save money on home utility bills, the brain and body have their own ways of saving energy. The metabolism can reduce the flow of nutrients to non-essential body functions—slowing down hair and nail growth, decreasing body temperature a fraction of a degree, or apportioning less fuel for immediate use, causing energy levels to decline. Also, because compared to survival, childbearing is a "want" and not a "must," both men and women can become less fertile. The brain and body may also decide to repair fewer cells, which may cause the body to ache or sustain injury more easily, or to redirect incoming fuel to pad the body's fat-storage areas.

Remember Kate, the Ironman competitor who couldn't understand why she gained sixty-five pounds when she was eating carefully and exercising fifteen to twenty hours per week? It turns out that Kate had metabolic syndrome that caused her to store fat from an early age. It's a very common condition—in fact, nearly 40 percent of U.S. adults in her demographic group suffer from metabolic syndrome—and it is potentially reversible with treatment. There is little scientific evidence, however, that dieting and exercise can "cure" this problem long-term. Rather, recent studies show that this syndrome can actually become more intense after dieting, just as Kate's weight came back in spite of a low caloric intake and high exercise expenditure. Her extreme calorie deficit only exacerbated her body's fear of deprivation

JUST THE FACTS

Scientific evidence shows that diet, exercise, and other lifestyle changes do not permanently correct hormone imbalances or the weight gain that these imbalances cause.

and amplified its weight-storing system, adding gasoline to the fire.

Once the weight defense system has been triggered, nothing—no diet, no eating plan, no "superfood," and no exercise regimen—can outsmart the disaster drills, backup plans, and fail-safes orchestrated by the brain and body.

DNA: GETTING TO THE ROOT OF THE PROBLEM

The propensity for metabolic malfunction exists in most of us, at least in one way or another. In those of us with prominent genetic vulnerabilities—people who are weight-prone rather than weight-resistant—it doesn't take much to disrupt our metabolism.

You can't really identify the precise root causes of metabolic malfunction without looking at DNA code. Research has shown that DNA affects insulin and leptin receptors, as well as factors like how much insulin, leptin, and POMC the body produces, and how sensitive the leptin receptors, MC3Rs, and MC4Rs are. To date, scientists have identified more than forty genetic variations and hundreds of specific genetic mutations that can contribute to weight-prone tendencies.[3] For example, some people may lack an enzyme required to prevent MSH from being too sticky. When MSH is too sticky, it glues itself to other molecules and becomes too bulky to fit easily into the "lock" that opens the MC4Rs (Door Four). Another variation may cause MSH to pick up an incorrect amino acid, changing its shape and preventing it from fitting into the receptors correctly. Some people experience other genetic vulnerabilities that slow down the pace of the communication pathway in their brain. And when *epigenetic changes* occur—when a person's original genes get modified over time—a pre-existing genetic tendency can surface or intensify. In theory, these genetic conditions can alter the brain receptors, making it more difficult for them to pick up hormonal signals.

Genetic variants affecting the metabolic feedback loop make some people more vulnerable to weight problems

---

3. B.M. Herrera, S. Keildson, C.M. Lindgren, "Genetics and epigenetics of obesity," *Maturitas* (May 2011), 69(1) doi: 10.1016/j.maturitas.2011.02.018 PMCID: PMC3213306: 41–49.

than others. When we compare the same locations on the DNA strands of people with and without weight problems, in fact, we often find that those without weight problems have built-in weight resistance. This might be because they have more than the normal amount of receptors, because their receptors are more sensitive to the signals, or because their receptors are resistant to shutting down—regardless, the end result is the same: they are more resistant to factors that can contribute to weight gain.

THANKS, MOM AND DAD

Many people experience weight challenges associated with their genetics. For example, a family history of type 2 diabetes or obesity is highly associated with a vulnerability to weight problems. In addition to genetic influences, children born at a low birth weight, children who went hungry in early life, children or adolescents who engaged in dieting at an early age, and those exposed to high levels of environmental obesogens are more vulnerable to adult overweight and obesity. This is also true for babies born to a mother with gestational diabetes. Babies born between 1940 and 1970 to women taking the drug DES (diethylstilbestrol) during pregnancy can also have an increased risk of future weight problems and increased diabetes risk. Tests from umbilical cord blood at birth show that alterations in the fat cell hormones leptin and adiponectin are associated with greater risk of overweight and obesity in the offspring by as early as age three to six years old.[4]

When nine-year-old Olivia came to see me, her body weight was already in a range that's considered extremely high, even for adults, and she reported an abnormally elevated appetite and significant fatigue. The tests I ran showed that due to her genetics and to unknown triggers (which were most probably encountered in the womb), Olivia had a severe case of insulin and leptin resistance. She had a number of glitches in her metabolic feedback loop.

It was difficult to manage Olivia's metabolic malfunctions because she was a child, and because, as in many cases of pediatric obesity and insulin resistance, her metabolic malfunctions were very strong. There are few medications that can be used by patients so young. Because of this, it was extremely difficult to medically treat Olivia and make an impact on correcting her metabolism, especially in the first few years I treated her. It was even more important than usual for her to get to bed

---

4. C.S. Mantzoros, S.L. Rifas-Shiman, et al., "Cord Blood Leptin and Adiponectin as Predictors of Adiposity in Children at 3 Years of Age: A Prospective Cohort Study," *Pediatrics* (February 2009), 123(2), doi: 10.1542/peds.2008-0343, PMCID: PMC2761663: 682–689.

on time and eat balanced meals and snacks, and the last thing a child or pre-teen wants to think about is healthy habits—taking medications, eating balanced meals, going to bed on time, and seeing doctors regularly. Her parents had to monitor her medication and supplement regimen to ensure she was on track. Her dad also took the time to join Olivia in physical activities she enjoyed, such as swimming, to help with her mobility.

In time, Olivia's health improved—and now, after years of work and in spite of the severity of her metabolic problem, we have finally begun to break through her powerful weight defenses. Her weight gain has not only stopped, it has begun a consistent downward trajectory. No amount of dieting and exercise could have fixed Olivia's Metabolic Storm. Her issues had to be addressed with a comprehensive program that included a regular schedule of supplements and targeted medication suitable for an adolescent.

FEAST OR FAMINE

A popular theory about what makes some of us more weight-prone than others is that some of us have remote or recent ancestors who experienced more famine than others. Although many people living in today's developed world give little thought to famines, they are among the oldest and most dangerous risks known to humankind. Where threats to our well-being are concerned, they rank up there with perils like lacking access to shelter and water, drowning, and being attacked by predators.

Although many of us use the phrase "dying from hunger" as a figure of speech, many of our forebears literally lived from feast to famine. The DNA of those who survived became encoded with data about how to endure food shortages. Our genes carry this knowledge forward from generation to generation, some experts believe. This survival mechanism protects us. It is so powerful that the brain and body of modern-day humans automatically assume that they are in danger unless hormonal signals convince them that the body is nutritionally safe and has an adequate, secure food supply and sufficient fat mass.

By studying the great famines throughout history, scientists have found that people whose ancestors survived famine conditions have a higher risk of developing weight problems than the descendants of ancestors whose food supply was never in peril. Gillian, whose ancestors were Irish farmers, is an excellent example of this. Obesity runs throughout her family tree, and when she was just a child, her concerned parents sent her to a diet clinic so she "wouldn't turn out like her obese relatives."

"I started dieting in second grade," Gillian reported. Her weight began to increase at an early age and continued to rise into adulthood, although she ate healthfully and stayed active. Eventually, at nearly 400 pounds, Gillian resorted to gastric bypass surgery. "But now," she said, "I've regained almost of the weight I lost since my surgery ten years ago."

Like many other people who struggle with weight problems, Gillian has a genetic vulnerability to obesity—her body's weight defense system, strongly influenced by her DNA, causes glitches in her metabolic feedback loop, and her past dieting and surgery have only amplified those glitches. No matter which tactic she uses, if she tries to lose weight her brain perceives it as deprivation, and it tells her body to store everything as fat for protection. Now, however, by identifying and treating her specific underlying glitches—which include metabolic syndrome and leptin resistance—she is finally beginning to address the problem at its root. This process will not take place overnight; it took years for Gillian to get to the point where she is now, and will take even more time for her metabolism to shift to a less "weight defensive" mode. But we are encouraged by the positive changes that are already beginning to take place in her health and weight trends.

WHAT CAN WE DO?

Research of the past two decades suggests that medically realigning the metabolic feedback loop is the key to long-term results when it comes to dealing with weight issues. It has also shown that hormonal irregularities that cause overweight and obesity cannot be corrected through any amount of willpower or control; these irregularities are caused by physiological problems, not behavior problems, and therefore they can only be solved through medical treatment. There are medications available today that can help most people correct metabolic malfunctions—and the more advancements we make in this area, the closer we are to revolutionizing the way society as a whole deals with weight problems. When it comes to overweight and obesity, science holds the answers.

CHAPTER 7

Science Holds the Answers

SO, IF DIET AND EXERCISE IS not an effective long-term solution to overweight and obesity, then what *is*? This is literally the $60 billion question—after all, that's what the diet industry is worth.

As we've previously discussed, science shows that weight problems are associated with complex underlying imbalances in the metabolic feedback loop. Accordingly, treatments that repair, reset, and realign the feedback loop are by far the most promising weight-loss options that exist today. And the good news is that scientists who are working on these types of solutions have made incredible progress in the past two decades; we are already benefitting from their discoveries and inventions, and can look forward to more innovative treatments on the way.

So, if science has the answers, why isn't anyone talking about them? In fact, researchers in this field *are* talking about the exciting new discoveries being made regarding the metabolism—it's just that most other people aren't privy to this information.

I have wondered why the science of metabolism and weight problems gets so little press. One reason may be that the growing diet industry, which permeates nearly every aspect of our daily life, drowns out the messages that science has to offer. People experience short-term results on diets, and they believe that the next one will work as well or better—and they think they haven't been successful in keeping off the weight because they didn't stick to the diet or it was just the wrong one, not because the idea of dieting is flawed. Another reason for the silence about metabolism's role in weight gain is that the pharmaceutical industry—the industry that is working on treatments I'm talking about—is dragging its feet. This is understandable: the AMA and a handful of other health organizations have accepted obesity as a medically treatable disease, but many others have not, so even if the pharmaceutical companies come up with safe, effective treatments, there's a good chance that few healthcare providers will prescribe them and no one will pay for them.

HISTORY REPEATS ITSELF

What I find truly fascinating about this area of medicine is that the most advanced and current scientific viewpoint of obesity is, in many ways, not new at all. In fact, as I explained in Chapter 5, it's actually close to one hundred years old. The leading endocrinologists and metabolic experts of the early 1900s recognized that diet and exercise were not a long-term "cure" for weight problems, and they believed the true solutions to addressing overweight and obesity would lie in hormonal treatments designed to realign the feedback loop. By the 1920s, these experts were writing that diet and exercise cures for obesity were already two decades outdated, and by the 1950s it was well established that diets slow metabolism down and therefore have significant limitations, even as a temporary solution. In the 1980s and '90s, several important metabolism-regulating hormones—amylin, leptin, adiponectin, and ghrelin—were discovered. And over the last decade, scientists who have studied the specific biochemical reasons why dieting causes metabolic slowdown have proven that diets leave a lasting fingerprint that promotes weight *regain*.

In Dr. Lisser's 1924 publication, "The Frequency of Endogenous Endocrine Obesity and Its Treatment By Glandular Therapy," he states:

I venture to predict that the supreme triumph
will come in the end from the isolation of hor-
mones specific for certain types of adiposity, just
as the pinnacle of diabetic research was reached
in insulin.

Lisser's prediction of future solutions based on the utilization of hormones and bioactive agents that are part of the metabolic feedback loop illustrates his great insight into metabolism and weight issues. Even with just the limited science that was available at the time, he understood that effective treatment of obesity would only be possible when the specific hormones involved in the metabolic process were identified. And it wasn't only Lisser who thought so: many prominent physicians of his time agreed. Dr. F.M. Pottenger, for example, had this to say in 1924:

A very large group of people suffer from obesity.
It was formerly thought that this was due to
overeating and lessened exercise. We now know,
however, that there are certain glands of inter-
nal secretion whose function influences greatly
the shape and size of the body.

Lisser's and Pottenger's contemporary, Dr. N.W. Janney, also believed that endocrine issues triggered obesity in most cases:

One or two decades ago it seemed sufficient to recognize exogenous obesity, due to overeating and underexercise, and endogenous obesity, usually vaguely relegated, to a "constitutional" or "familial" tendency . . . With accumulation of knowledge of the ductless glands, it has, however, become a certainty that an endocrine etiologic factor underlies the development of overweight in most cases, as Dr. Lisser's timely paper emphasizes.

Lisser and his colleagues honed in on the concept of an underlying metabolic problem being the root cause of obesity, and their vision of a cure that focused on hormonal regulation of the fat tissue was incredibly insightful. But due to the complexity of this task, it has taken scientists nearly one hundred years to map out the pathophysiology (abnormal physiology) of these underlying causes of obesity and translate it into viable potential treatments.

OBESITY UNDER THE MICROSCOPE

During this ninety-year absence of effective medical treatment, the diet industry has blossomed into what it is today, even as diet and exercise studies have been repeated over and over again with the same results: a lack of long-term effectiveness, slowing of the metabolic rate, and a metabolic fingerprint that encourages weight regain. It's as though we believe if we conduct enough studies, the results will be different. What if we had funneled those resources into exploring novel concepts and potential treatments?

Results of today's clinical lab tests reflect that weight problems are driven by metabolic problems. My patients initially report symptoms of appetite irregularity, fatigue, and weight-loss resistance, and they show abnormal levels and functions in many aspects of their metabolic feedback loops. Typical lab results indicate low leptin levels, low adiponectin, low MSH levels, excessive ghrelin, insulin resistance and/or leptin resistance. The ability to objectively diagnose metabolic problems that cause obesity through lab testing is critical. If weight problems are diagnosed medically, the treatment focus shifts from merely targeting the weight-related symptoms by prescribing a diet or exercise plan and moves toward one of treating the underlying metabolic malfunction itself.

While the availability of clinical tests has improved dramatically over the past decade, we still cannot test a patient's genes to identify genetic vulnerabilities—the new FTO gene associated with obesity, for example—nor can we conduct chromosome analysis that would clarify where the most vulnerable hereditary areas are along the metabolic feedback loop. However, we *can* improve the function of the metabolic feedback loop through individualized medical treatments. Almost one hundred years after first being recognized by Lisser as the "supreme triumph" of obesity treatment, the dream of pinpointing the underlying hormonal causes of weight gain and using medications to address them can finally become a reality.

THE COCKTAIL APPROACH

The role of medications is just beginning to be better understood. Metabolic problems are complex, so each patient needs a customized plan—a "cocktail" approach that combines sophisticated medications to attack multiple glitches along the feedback loop. In some cases the plan involves bariatric surgery, which, like medication, often has metabolic impact.

A recent article published in *Disease Models & Mechanisms* emphasizes that combination treatment is the most promising strategy for addressing weight problems:[1]

---

1. R.J. Rodgers, M.H. Tschöp, J.P.H. Wilding, "Anti-obesity drugs: past, present and future," *Disease Models & Mechanisms* (September 2012), 5(5), doi: 10.1242/dmm.009621, PMCID: PMC3424459: 621–626.

To succeed in developing drugs that control body weight to the extent seen following surgical intervention, it seems obvious that a new paradigm is needed. In future, this polytherapeutic strategy could possibly rival surgery in terms of efficacy, safety and sustainability of weight loss.

The goal of any medical treatment should be to address what's causing the problem, not merely to mask the symptoms. If you had a headache and it kept coming back, wouldn't you rather try to find out why than simply take aspirin day after day as a temporary fix? Wouldn't you wonder what was causing the headache to recur? Weight problems are no different.

PHARMACOLOGY PIPELINE

Medical treatment is a way of bridging gaps in the metabolic feedback loop and restoring the flow of signals. Once patients have made sufficient progress and their system returns to normalcy, medications can be gradually withdrawn. Several medications have the potential to favorably impact the metabolic pathways. Next, we'll discuss some of those medications.

Metformin

Metformin, one of the oldest medications used to correct glitches in the metabolic pathway was discovered in the 1920s, and is still the most widely prescribed medication for type 2 diabetes today. It acts as a gatekeeper, regulating the pace at which the liver releases glucose between meals so there are no sudden surges of glucose into the bloodstream.

Synthetic Hormones

Newer medications designed to address issues in the metabolic pathway include synthetic forms of the hormones involved. *Incretin mimetics*, synthetic hormones that were introduced to the market in 2005, mimic GLP-1, the hormone that is normally produced in the intestine. Like GLP-1, incretin mimetics help the brain see the nutrition in our food, regulate the pace at which food moves through our stomach and small intestine, and the pace at which nutrients are absorbed into the bloodstream. They also regulate glucagon levels, and thus the rate at which glucose is released from the liver during periods of fasting. They improve cardiometabolic indicators, such as blood pressure and cholesterol levels, as well as insulin sensitivity and visceral fat levels and they have a favorable impact on ghrelin, NPY, and AGRP. In diabetics, incretin mimetics help the pancreas match the blood sugar with the appropriate amount of insulin by stimulating growth of new insulin-producing beta cells to replace some of those that no longer function.

A synthetic form of the hormone *amylin* was released in 2005. It improves insulin sensitivity and leptin sensitivity, allowing diabetic patients to use less insulin to control their blood sugar levels, and, similar to incretin mimetics, it regulates the pace of glucagon release. Amylin has a synergistic action with leptin: it augments the leptin signal in the brain, more clearly informing the brain of the body's weight status. In doing so, it reduces NPY and AGRP levels at Door One of the central metabolic pathway.

DPP-4 inhibitors, first released in 2006, can be used to inhibit the body's ability to break down GLP-1, thereby prolonging the effects of the GLP-1 the body produces on its own.

Other Metabolic Pathway Modifiers

The medication *topiramate* was discovered in 1979 and has been on the U.S. market since 1996. Originally developed to help prevent migraine headaches, topiramate's effect upon weight regulation has now been studied for many years. Although the exact mechanisms of its action are unknown, it is thought that its effectiveness is primarily due to its favorable impact on NPY activity at Door One in the central metabolic pathway.

Bupropion increases activity at Door Two of the central metabolic pathway and production of the hormone MSH. It is a component of two new obesity medications that are in development: *Contrave*, which consists of bupropion and a medication called naltrexone, which augments bupropion's metabolic action; and *Empatic*, which combines bupropion with zonisamide, a medication that is similar to topiramate. Contrave and Empatic are anticipated to be released within the next two years. *Lorcaserin*, a medication released in 2013, also activates Door 2, but via a different mechanism.

Phentermine, an appetite blocker, and *orlistat*, a fat-absorption blocker, are also used in weight regulation, but they mainly focus on the lowering of food intake or lowering of food absorption rather than on a specific metabolic action, making them some of the least sophisticated medications in the group.

NEWER INVENTIONS ON THE HORIZON

The next decade will be very exciting for healthcare providers and patients as new treatment options become available. Researchers are developing synthetic versions of other hormones and chemicals that help to regulate the metabolic feedback loop—MSH, adiponectin, leptin, a leptin/amylin combination, oxyntomodulin, and PYY— as well as blockers and supporters of specific functions along the feedback loop. Others have developed an immunization that reduces elevated ghrelin, and still others are studying new ways to stimulate "brown fat," which is highly metabolically active.

In combination with the medications that are already on the market, these promising treatments still in development may address most of the common glitches in the metabolic pathway. Genetic testing is also on the horizon, and will eventually be useful in making diagnoses. As science continues to progress—and it's happening at an amazingly fast pace—our ability to clinically measure the body's metabolic hormones and apply more effective treatment will only increase.

BARIATRIC SURGERY

Many physicians today are promoting bariatric surgeries, such as gastric bypass, vertical sleeve, and lap band, as a way to not only to lose weight but also reverse diabetes. These surgeries do have *some* benefits: they produce some of the most impressive weight-loss rates of any treatment available, and although most people experience weight regain post-op, they usually don't regain *all* of the weight lost. The Vertical Sleeve Gastroplasty (VSG) and Roux-en-Y gastric bypass surgery (RYGB) have even been shown to favorably alter some of the hormones disrupted by both original metabolic problems and prior diets. However, surgery often doesn't really reverse the underlying cause of the weight problem, and it can eventually impact the metabolism like a diet, triggering the body's weight defense system and leading to weight regain.

Many of my patients who have undergone bariatric procedures have come to me for help with weight regain or blood sugar regulation issues in the months or years following their surgery. In the short term, many of them lost a great deal of weight—100, 150, or even 200 pounds within a couple of years—especially those who had a VSG or Roux-en-Y gastric bypass procedure. And the surgery does, in fact, bump many patients out of diabetes and back into pre-diabetes, insulin resistance, or even normal status in some cases. In the majority of these cases, however, at least a portion of the lost weight is eventually regained.

The RYGB is both a restrictive and absorptive surgery, meaning it reduces the size of the stomach and blocks the absorption of certain nutrients from the small intestine into the bloodstream. On the other hand, the VSG or "sleeve" procedure is a purely restrictive surgery that reduces the size of the stomach but does not interfere with nutrient absorption. The sleeve permanently removes the portion of the stomach that secretes ghrelin (the anti-metabolism hormone), so this can be a very effective solution for some patients. Both the VSG and RYGB have been shown to improve the function of many of the incretins (hormones from the lower intestine) within days after surgery.

In contrast to the VSG and RYBG, most long-term studies have shown lap band surgery to be largely unsuccessful. This procedure is restrictive—it shrinks the stomach's capacity—but unlike VSG, it does not appear to significantly improve pre-existing hormonal imbalances. Rather, it may have an extreme-diet effect, potentially leading to very high ghrelin levels and, subsequently, considerable rebound weight gain.

Regardless of which surgery is performed—VSG, RYBG, or lap band—I have found that medically monitoring patients afterward for recurrence of hormone malfunctions related to their original metabolic problem or the impact of the surgery itself improves post-surgical response. Physicians routinely advise all bariatric surgery patients to stay on a low-calorie diet and exercise for an hour most days for the rest of their lives. But dieting after bariatric surgery can backfire over the long term, just like any other diet. Bariatric surgery can *improve* incretin function short term, but it doesn't *cure* the underlying metabolic problem—which means that dieting post-surgery can still set off your body's weight defense system. Many patients eventually develop Diet Fog and their Metabolic Storm returns, causing them to regain a significant amount of weight and, in some cases, triggering a return to diabetes.

In order to achieve optimal results, it's helpful to assess a patient's metabolic problem *prior* to surgery. While some people may indeed need surgery, others don't. There are nonsurgical medical options that may be effective. And scientific studies of metabolism show us that improving hormone function permanently is necessary for long-term success. Ultimately, solving lifelong metabolic issues requires an individualized approach, and it can't happen overnight. That said, the majority of my patients do well with medical treatment.

REVERSING DIABESITY: JANET'S STORY

When Janet, age fifty, first came to visit me, she was seriously obese. She was so afraid to gain weight that she barely ate anything—but in spite of this, she kept gaining. Among her various health problems, I discovered that Janet had undiagnosed type 2 diabetes. When we met, she was on so many medications that she could hardly keep her eyes open. She had run marathons when she was younger, but by the time she reached me she could barely get up off of the couch. I was shocked when she told me, "I want to be a competitive swimmer."

Once we began medical treatment, Janet's hormonal settings gradually began to change. Within several months of adjusting medications, eating more regularly, and beginning to address her metabolic problems, Janet's health had markedly improved. She was feeling much better. Although her body was initially resistant to weight loss, we worked on building her fitness while fueling each workout well so that her body's weight defenses would not activate. Within three years, in line with her goals, Janet actually entered her first swim competition. Over the next couple of years, changes in medication and additional correction of her underlying metabolic problems eventually led to steady weight loss.

Today, Janet has reached a normal weight and body fat percentage, and she no longer has diabetes or even pre-diabetes. She has been free of diabetes for three years and has maintained a normal body weight for the past two years—and she's done so while eating more regularly than she ever had before we began treatment. She has met her goal of swimming competitively, and she now dreams of one day swimming the English Channel. Recovery didn't happen overnight for Janet, but after years of consistent treatment, she has experienced remarkable improvements in her health.

A SCIENTIFIC TREATMENT APPROACH

In my more than twenty-five years of practice, I've never had a single patient develop diabetes under my care—including those who were at high risk for having diabetes, and those who already had pre-diabetes, or insulin resistance when they first came to see me. While it's nice to celebrate weight loss, as a physician I'm most interested in what is going on with blood pressure, cholesterol, blood sugar, fatty liver, and other conditions. My first priority is always health. What's on the inside is what is most important.

I have adopted a strategy for helping patients achieve better metabolic function that is certainly more rewarding than the strategy I employed when I first approached this problem twenty years ago with a "calories in, calories out" mindset. This process is straightforward: apply known science and available tools; obtain objective testing through lab work; collect in-depth patient history; and talk with and listen to the patient. Then I can see what the landscape shows in terms of opportunity to adjust hormonal misalignments in both hormonal levels and their reception throughout the body. The goal is to reconnect and strengthen the communication feedback loop between my patient's brain and body to gain metabolic balance. Sometimes this involves adjusting exercise programs or backing off on exercise altogether for a while. Other times it may involve eating a more balanced diet, eating meals and snacks more frequently, or going to bed earlier. In most cases, it includes finding the most appropriate medications to cast, splint, support, and close the gaps that fragment the metabolic feedback loop to restore communication throughout the loop.

When this individualized approach is successful, weight maintenance gradually becomes easier, weight reduction becomes possible, and appetite regulation eventually becomes easy and natural—and regardless of changes in body weight, health problems that were associated with the underlying metabolic issues nearly always improve. In addition, energy levels and overall quality of life usually improve.

It's important to understand that this process is not a cakewalk for a physician or a patient. It takes patience, careful monitoring, and juggling variables to support the body through nourishment, sleep, and consistent medical treatment. Weight problems are most often a chronic medical condition, and treatment is a *process*. So treatment won't look like taking a course of antibiotics for a sinus infection. Rather, it will be an ongoing process of evaluation and treatment, requiring frequent monitoring and updating.

Step 1: Identifying the Problem

There are usually two issues at play when treating a weight problem—the original metabolic problem (the

JUST THE FACTS

Good health habits apply to everyone at any weight. Taking care of ourselves is a personal responsibility.

• Eat nutritious foods
• Be physically active
• Get enough sleep

Metabolic Storm) and the secondary effects caused by prolonged dieting and/or excessive exercise (Diet Fog). Although we cannot yet clinically test for every hormone in the body, an objective workup provides valuable information that reveals the chessboard, so to speak, on which we are playing—allowing us to see where kinks and gaps in the metabolic pathway are likely blocking hormonal signals from getting through to the brain and back. I, as the physician, am on one side of the chessboard, and the patient's cagey weight defense system is on the other, trying to outsmart us. Once we have the necessary information, we then determine which moves we should make to treat the affected areas of the pathway, always aiming to be one step ahead of our opponent.

Step 2: Make the Body Feel Nutritionally Secure

Regardless of whether lab results suggest Diet Fog (low leptin, low insulin, and usually high ghrelin) or point to the original metabolic problem (which varies among patients, but usually results in the brain and body perceiving that fuel is scarce or fat mass is too low), you must first shut down the body's weight defense system before you can make any progress at all.

When it comes to healing metabolic issues, nutritional eating and well-fueled exercise have many benefits, but it's important to shift our thinking about food and exercise from weight goals to *health* goals. We do have weight goals, but the thinking and behavior that support those goals should not be based on deprivation or control. We don't want to further exacerbate the problems of an already weak, fragmented metabolic feedback loop by making the body feel deprived. So, fueling consistently, fueling exercise well, and avoiding dietary rigidity are critical to making the body feel nutritionally secure. Adequate sleep is also important, because metabolic hormone balancing primarily occurs when we are asleep.

These health-based principles and recommendations are exactly the same as the ones I provide to patients who are trying to recover metabolically and physically from anorexia. The goal is to restore their metabolic function and balance their weight to a healthy range. Patients who tell me they struggle with binge eating, emotional eating, stress eating, compulsive overeating, or boredom eating think they are dealing with behavioral issues, but what they are really dealing with are biological symptoms. Although weight problems are certainly not psychological, stress can physiologically divert metabolic activity away from the appetite and metabolism receptors, which can contribute to glitches in the central metabolic pathway. When we realign the malfunctioning hormones, the biology is restored to normal, and the issues considered "bad behaviors" cease to be a problem.

Step 3: A New View on Fueling and Sleep
Prioritize Eating

This is the most counterintuitive principal, and the one that my new patients are most surprised to hear—but prioritizing eating is key to successful treatment. If you're going to deactivate your weight defense system, your body needs to know that it can trust you to feed it. So put self-nourishment at the top of your to-do list. Plan when and how you *will* nourish yourself rather than planning when and how you will *not* nourish yourself. Have conversations with yourself about *eating* rather than *not eating*. Your brain and body are listening. If you nourish yourself as you say you will, in time they will learn to trust you. This means eating breakfast within an hour of waking and then eating every few hours throughout the day to fuel your body. Alternate meals and snacks, and include all food groups. Don't go hungry.

✈ *Eat for Health*

Rather than associating food with weight, your new nutritional goal is to *not* cut calories, stick to a plan, or eat (or not eat) a certain kind of food. I realize this sounds crazy to most people who are used to being told that dieting is mandatory for weight loss, and that it's very difficult for most people to transition from a life of dieting to a life without diets. Many patients I see are still dieting and have a diet mentality about food, even if they think they do not. I work with dietitians, and together we help patients understand what "not dieting" really means.

Your new goal is to nourish your brain and body with balanced meals and snacks so reliably throughout the day that they stop transmitting starvation signals. As the starvation signaling dies down, important changes will begin to take place: you will think more clearly, and your mood and energy will improve. With medical assistance, your metabolism will begin to repair and restore itself, and instead of Diet Fog, the Metabolic Storm, and weight gain, you will begin to experience the benefits of healthy fuel burning.

Change Your Mindset

All foods provide us with fuel. In that sense—and because you now understand that hormonal imbalances, not food, are what cause your weight problem—there are no good or bad foods. The minute you start being rigid and making rules, you will either gravitate to "off-limits" foods more than ever before or you'll activate your body's weight defense system, causing your metabolism to shut down.

Fuel Yourself Consistently and Steadily

Eat three balanced meals every day, plus two to four snacks, so you never deprive your brain and body of fuel. This translates into eating every three hours or so. If you do not adequately fuel your brain, it will slow your metabolism to protect itself. This means you cannot afford to skip any meals. Yes, people with normal metabolisms may occasionally skip meals, but they can get away with it because their body doesn't fear starvation. Their weight defense system isn't ready to engage at any moment the way yours is. And don't forget to eat before exercise to provide your body with fuel, and immediately after exercise to restore your muscles' carbohydrate (glycogen) stores for your next workout.

Eat from All Three Macronutrient Groups at Each Meal

Everyone feels better if they eat from all food groups. Carbs are the brain and body's primary source of fuel, and fat and protein, in addition to having many other beneficial functions, help to regulate the pace of digestion. You need all of these macronutrients to be healthy and to offset the effects of your underlying hormonal malfunctions. Whenever possible, vary your sources of macronutrients while emphasizing foods that provide steady nutrition and support health. For example, three to five servings of whole grains daily is associated with reduced risk of diabetes, cardiovascular disease, and weight gain.[2]

Eat to Feel Good

Vegan, pescatarian, omnivore—all of these eating choices are fine, as long as they're driven by what makes you feel your best rather than by some diet fad or false belief that they will solve your weight problem.

Eat for Enjoyment

Eating for enjoyment is healthy. This is often a challenge for people who have lived a life of rigid dieting, control,

---

2. E.Q. Ye, S.A. Chacko, et al., "Greater whole-grain intake is associated with lower risk of type 2 diabetes, cardiovascular disease, and weight gain," *Journal of Nutriton* (July 2012),142(7), doi: 10.3945/jn.111.155325: 1304-1313.

and deprivation. People who take time to enjoy food as part of their culture appear to have healthier metabolisms than most Americans. For example, the French and Italians fall much lower than Americans do in obesity rankings. And the Spanish eat very late at night—a supposed no-no in this country—and yet their obesity levels are far below ours. Traditionally, these other cultures don't have a lot of strict rules about eating. Eating supports their lifestyle—it doesn't control it. So, if you want some ice cream, have some and enjoy it.

⚡ *Get Adequate Sleep*

Sleep is critical for health, metabolism, and weight regulation. It provides recovery from the day's activities, and it reboots your entire system so your body is prepared for the demands of the next day. During sleep, the body regenerates muscle mass, builds bones and lean mass, and many important hormones that regulate metabolism are secreted throughout the night. Optimal sleep improves metabolism, energy, and mood.

The anti-metabolism hormone ghrelin is secreted primarily between midnight and 2 a.m., and the pro-metabolism hormone leptin is usually secreted between 2 and 4 a.m. Falling asleep well before these hormones secrete is optimal for healthy hormone balance. Your hormone secretion schedule may change based on when you eat breakfast and when you eat the last meal of your day, however. If you have a job that requires an early morning wake time, it's best to have breakfast early. This will encourage your hormone cycles to complete earlier in the night, before you wake up. When hormone cycles become disrupted or if sleep duration is under seven hours, the result is usually a higher ghrelin response and a lower leptin response. Basically, inadequate sleep can contribute to weight gain and weight-loss resistance, especially in overweight and obese patients.

HOW DOES THE SCIENCE WORK IN REAL LIFE?

The following examples show what happens when medical treatment based on science is combined with a non-diet approach.

JANET

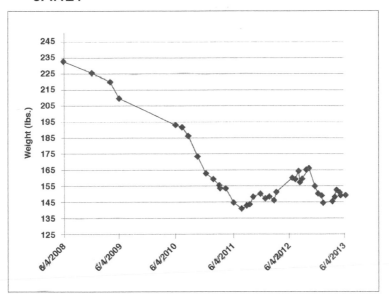

Janet used to run marathons but had gradually become seriously obese over a number of years when she was placed on medications for depression. When I first saw her, she was unaware that she had type 2 diabetes. Eventually, her metabolism began to adjust, and her weight began to decrease. Janet has since been able to reach a normal body weight and body fat percentage. Her diabetes has been gone for three years now, and she does not have pre-diabetes. Like all of my patients, these results were achieved not by dieting but by correcting underlying metabolic malfunctions.

LILLY

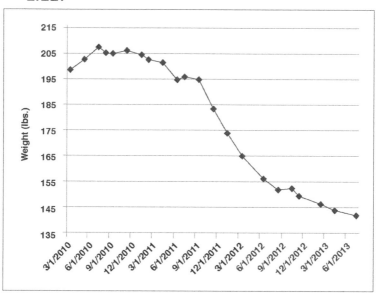

Lilly had weight problems most of her life. She had a history of extreme dieting, and her weight issues increased when she began to attend grad school. It took about a year to reverse her Diet Fog and then control her leptin resistance—but in the past two years, her blood tests have shown improvement and her body weight has gradually and persistently dropped. Solely through realigning her metabolic feedback loop, Lilly's weight has been brought down to a normal range.

LAUREN

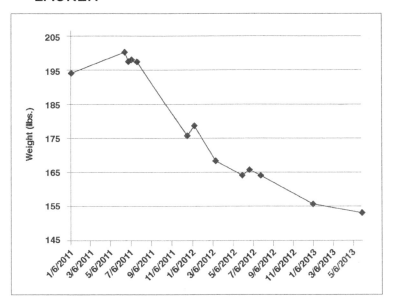

Lauren, a college student and professional cyclist, had a history of struggling with her weight. In spite of her heavy exercise load, she dieted constantly in an attempt to keep her weight from climbing. Before I met her, she had suffered an injury and had been treated with steroids, which contributed to rapid weight gain. Lauren's blood test showed significant Diet Fog. She had an initial weight increase while we dismantled her extreme dieting behavior, which was very frustrating for her, but once the Diet Fog cleared and we could address the underlying cause of her weight problem—insulin resistance—Lauren experienced steady weight loss. She is now maintaining a normal weight range, fueling her body well, and successfully competing again.

MADDY

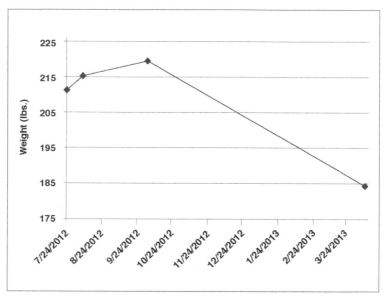

Before seeing me, Maddy, age seventeen, had battled weight problems since early childhood. Her mother was very concerned because Maddy was doing everything "right" but getting nowhere. Finally, Maddy's mother brought her to see me. Maddy's lab tests showed extreme Diet Fog—and after she stopped exercising and started eating foods that she loved for the first time in her life, we identified the underlying problem: insulin resistance. With medical treatment, Maddy's weight has declined at a steady pace, and based on her lab work and progress so far, I am confident it will continue to do so.

RACHAEL

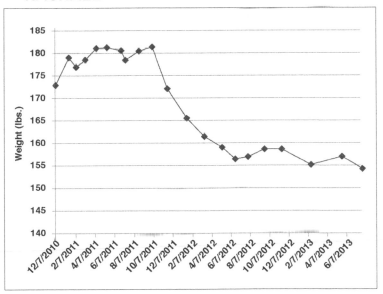

Before coming to see me, Rachael strictly followed a 1,200- to 1,400-calorie diet. A typical meal was chicken breast, salad, and steamed vegetables. Once a day she might allow herself a scoop of brown rice—but no dessert. She also exercised heavily—often two to three hours a day, participating in a boot camp program or training for a triathlon. Still, she was overweight, and her weight was steadily increasing in spite of her efforts.

Today, Rachael eats nutritious food, but she doesn't count calories or restrict her eating. In fact, she eats mashed potatoes, bread, maple bars, and chocolate cake when she wants to—foods that were strictly off limits for her for years. Rachel did not exercise during most of her treatment—especially at first, so that her metabolism could recover from Diet Fog—but she still lost a significant amount of weight.

DIANNE

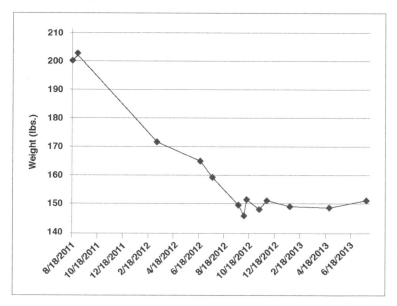

Dianne, 42, started dieting at age 12. She had some short-term success losing weight through dieting but began to gain rapidly after quitting smoking and going through a stressful move. Dianne joined a gym, worked out regularly, watched what she ate and avoided carbohydrates. "I have tried everything! I'm in better shape than ever but now I'm heavier than I've ever been," Dianne said with exasperation. Smoking lowers the metabolism blocker, NPY. When Dianne stopped smoking her metabolic problems became more difficult to manage. Fortunately, she responded to a minimal amount of medication which reversed her underlying metabolic dysfunction.

DAVID

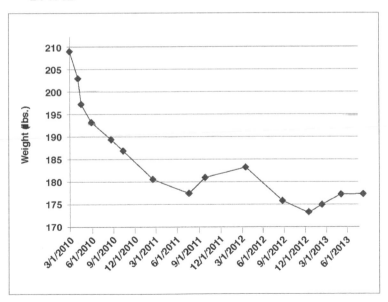

David, 58, came to see me to find out why he couldn't lose weight and why he felt "off." I found he had full-blown type 2 diabetes and metabolic syndrome. David had no idea he had these conditions or that his weight was a symptom of a much bigger underlying problem. He had high blood pressure, high cholesterol with plaque in his arteries, and his HBA1C was 8.8 (normal is 4.8-5.6). Now David is full of energy. His HBA1C is 5.9 and his blood pressure and cholesterol are in the lowest risk ranges.

BILL

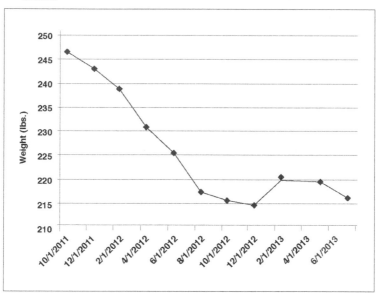

Bill, six feet tall and 52 years old, came into my office with a stubborn weight problem and intense sugar cravings. I found that his weight problem was a symptom of a deeper medical issue. He had undiagnosed metabolic syndrome with insulin resistance and pre-diabetes, high cholesterol and LDL particles, and increased abdominal fat. Bill now has normal blood sugar levels, normal cholesterol and LDL levels, and normal blood pressure. Although his weight loss is moderate in terms of pounds, Bill's body composition has improved significantly. We used a cocktail of medication to reverse Bill's stubborn metabolic dysfunction. He is doing so well that we are going to taper off some of the medications soon.

DANA

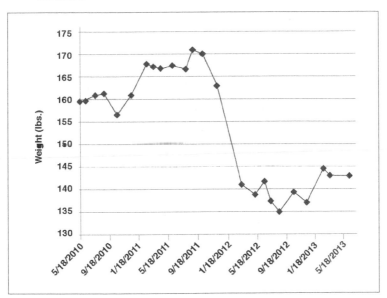

Dana, who is now 19 years old, first came to me as an adolescent after attending a diet boot camp to lose weight. She lost weight rapidly at the camp but eventually the weight began to creep back even though she was counting every calorie and exercising regularly. I found that Dana was in extreme Diet Fog. She was chronically tired, her menstrual cycles had stopped, she suffered several stress fractures and had low bone density. Dana's lab work showed that she had what essentially looked like anorexia caused by her diet and exercise program. It took about a year for her to come out of Diet Fog. The best we could do was to minimize the gain and stabilize her weight until, by eating regularly and abstaining from exercise, she came out of the Diet Fog. At that point, Dana's labs showed that insulin resistance was the root cause of her weight problem. After treating and reversing the insulin resistance, Dana's metabolism works normally. She has tapered off of insulin resistance treatment and remains on only a small amount of medical support—which will soon not be needed. The most important fact is that when she first came to my office Dana was literally starving and counting every calorie while gaining weight. Now she is eating freely, far more nourished, and has a stable weight and metabolism.

BETTY

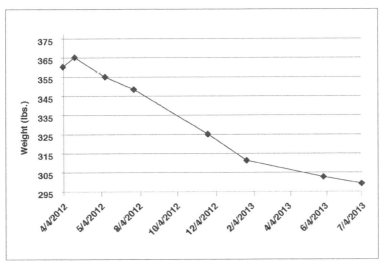

Betty, 65, suffered from knee arthritis and was unable to walk without a cane. She wanted more than anything to be able to play with her grandkids and have enough stamina to get through the day. Betty reported a long standing history of obesity. She said, "When I was just 14, I had to starve myself to get my weight to go down at all." She had irregular hunger and satiety symptoms, often finding herself waking up in the middle of the night hungry. I found Betty had metabolic syndrome with high cholesterol, high blood pressure and pre-diabetes. Betty's excess weight was a symptom of underlying metabolic dysfunction. By focusing on regular eating, not dieting and medically treating the underlying metabolic problems, Betty's health issues have finally begun to significantly resolve, her symptoms have disappeared and her weight is steadily declining. She is enjoying time with her grandchildren and has much more stamina.

BACK TO NORMAL

As patients' metabolisms heal, their appetite, tastes, cravings, hunger-related sensations, and feelings of satisfaction normalize. One patient, Kay, shared with me, "I can't overstate how free I feel. Is this what normal people do? I feel like a normal human being for the first time. I can walk into the kitchen at work and candy doesn't call. I can get through the day. I don't feel deprivation around eating."

The body stops gaining weight when the metabolic signals make their way to the MC4Rs at Door Four of the metabolic pathway. And as the metabolism stabilizes, patients begin to lose weight automatically. When the metabolism normalizes, issues with blood pressure, cholesterol, or glucose usually improve significantly as well, even when no weight is lost.

MAKING PROGRESS AFTER 27 YEARS: CLAUDIA'S STORY

"Twenty-seven years ago I gained one hundred pounds in one year, even though I didn't change my diet or exercise," Claudia told me the first time we met. "I have been trying to figure out how to lose that weight ever since."

She tried various diets with no success, including one extreme diet, before deciding to go to one of the most prominent medical centers in the U.S. Claudia was shocked and dismayed when the head of the center's Division of Endocrinology, Diabetes, Metabolism, and Nutrition advised: "If you hire a personal trainer to work with you twice a week for forty-five minutes of isometric exercise and follow a 1,400 calorie diet, I have no doubt that you will lose four pounds per month." Claudia knew very well from experience that this advice wasn't going to solve her weight issues—she had tried even more extreme measures than this in the past, and none of them had worked.

When Claudia came to me, I initially saw metabolic problems including Diet Fog, and soon after that, I also discovered that she had leptin resistance. Gradually it became clear that she had an MC4R (Door Four) malfunction. It was also evident that, prior to her weight increase, she had been given a medication that disrupted a section of her metabolic pathway, which was probably what triggered her sudden weight gain. After all those years of failed diets, and after another year of treatment with me, Claudia has finally begun to make progress on weight loss and metabolic rebalancing through medical treatment—

and without dieting. The strategies we've implemented are working slowly and steadily, and we hope to be able to navigate an effective treatment for the long term.

THE KNOWLEDGE EXPLOSION

The science of obesity and metabolism is one of the most exciting fields of medicine today; it is virtually exploding with promising new discoveries and inventions. Dr. Lisser's one-hundred-year-old dream is finally becoming a reality. We are gaining knowledge and strategies that can begin to solve our country's weight issues. With the discoveries of numerous hormones that regulate the metabolic feedback loop and the inventions of medications that can restore normal metabolic function, we are well on our way to making the Diabesity Epidemic something of the past.

Dieting offers little chance of long-term success because it does not "cure" the underlying cause of most people's weight problems. People stop dieting because diets stop working. Patients don't fail diets—diets fail them.

CONCLUSION

Science Never Sleeps

WHEN WE CONSIDER HOW we as a society view weight problems, we are living in medieval times—which is why I'm so thrilled to bring you up to date on what scientists have discovered and what that means for people who are dealing with overweight and obesity.

We now know that metabolism is regulated by a complex feedback loop with the brain as the CEO and the hormones as the messengers, and we have learned that glitches can occur along this feedback loop, impairing metabolism, promoting fat storage, and often causing the appetite to increase—the Metabolic Storm. We also know that there are strong genetic influences that increase weight-prone tendencies, and that in genetically vulnerable people, glitches can be triggered by environmental factors such as dieting (especially in childhood), sleep deprivation, certain medications, and endocrine-disrupting obesogens. These glitches are not within a person's control—they are a medical problem, and should be treated as such.

For nearly one hundred years, scientists have proven that diets don't "cure" overweight and obesity—and, worse, that they actually aggravate the problem by slowing metabolism and leaving a lasting fingerprint that encourages weight regain. According to multiple studies, even exercise cannot prevent this slowdown.

Healthcare providers, trainers, friends, family, and co-workers who recommend diets are well-meaning—but they often fail to realize that while dieting may seem to work in the short term, long-term maintenance of weight lost through dieting is generally unrealistic.

It has been nearly a century since physicians and scientists first began to explore the metabolic causes and potential treatments of obesity. We have finally discovered and isolated numerous hormone messengers and brain components involved in metabolism and proven their actions and interactions, uncovering the peripheral and central metabolic pathways. We now have treatments available to realign the metabolic feedback loop, with promising advances on the horizon. Science is catching up to the impressive insight of those endocrinologists of the 1920s who challenged the thinking of their time—and we are now making real progress in this area of medicine.

What we have learned from studying weight problems and metabolism is that the perceptions many of us have of people confronted with overweight and obesity are often *mis*perceptions. Weight and health are not necessarily related: you can be healthy or fit at any weight, and unhealthy or unfit at any weight. And while it's nice to celebrate weight loss, it's what's on the inside that is most important.

An obese person's brain is essentially blind to the excess weight the body is carrying, and this can lead to preoccupation with food and impaired satisfaction after eating. So, like the excess weight itself, increased appetite is a symptom of an underlying problem. That's why simply dieting or using discipline to control food intake does not fix the problem long-term.

Medical conditions are associated with specific symptoms and abnormal test findings, and are addressed with medical treatment. Based on that definition, obesity is a medical condition. If the thyroid is not functioning normally, we take thyroid hormones to stay in optimal ranges. If we have an infection, we use antibiotics to eradicate it. If we have a tumor, we perform surgery or chemotherapy to reduce its size. So when it comes to overweight and obesity, why don't we apply the same perspective?

Today, science offers so much hope for people experiencing weight problems. Over the next decade, scientists will be busy refining more synthetic hormones and agents that block or accentuate hormone action, and will be coming up with other strategies that retrain and normalize metabolic function.

The more we know about how the metabolism works, the more obvious it is that weight problems are medical problems and they are not anyone's fault. Most patients can already benefit from treatments that exist today—but there is still progress to be made.

Thankfully for us, science never sleeps.

End Notes

Chapter 5 Timeline Sources:

Wikipedia.org, *History of Diabetes,* http://en.wikipedia.org/wiki/History_of_diabetes (July 2013).

D.V. Fenby, "Heat: Its measurement from Galileo to Lavoisier,"*Pure and Applied Chemistry* (1987), Vol. 59, No. 1: 91—100.

Wikipedia.org, *Body Mass Index,* http://en.wikipedia.org/wiki/Body_mass_index.

E.A.M Gale, "Timeline 1900-1950," Diapedia (July 27, 2013), 1104709121 Rev. No. 7.

A. Mazur, "Why were 'starvation diets' promoted for diabetes in the pre-insulin period?," *Nutrition Journal* (2011), 10:23, doi: 10.1186/1475-2891-10-23.

Wikipedia.org, *Lulu Hunt Peters*, http://en.wikipedia. org/wiki/Lulu_Hunt_Peters.

B.W. McGuinness, "Melanocyte-Stimulating Hormone: A Clinical And Laboratory Study," *Annals of the New York Academy of Sciences* (December 15, 2006), DOI: 10.1111/ j.1749-6632.1963.tb42921.x.

Nobelprize.org, *The Discovery of Insulin*, http://www. nobelprize.org/educational/medicine/insulin/discovery-insulin.html.

Wikipedia.org, *Metformin*, http://en.wikipedia.org/wiki/ Metformin.

N.R. Gosmanov, A.R. Gosmanov, J.E. Gerich, *Glucagon Physiology*, Endotext.org (February 4, 2011), http://www. endotext.org/diabetes/diabetes2/diabetes2.html.

H. Lisser, "The Frequency Of Endogenous Endocrine Obesity And Its Treatment By Glandular Therapy," *California and Western Medicine* (October 1924), Vol. XXII, No. 10: 509-514.

A. Majid, *Integrated Insulin and Toxic Metal Reductions for Coronary Heart Disease*, Majidaliacademy.org, http:// www.majidaliacademy.org/insulin_reduction.htm.

Glucagon.com, *The Incretin Effect*, Glucagon.com, http://www.glucagon.com/incretineffect.html. M. Sattley, "The History of Diabetes," *Diabetes Health* (November 1996).

Wikipedia.org, *NPH Insulin*, http://en.wikipedia.org/wiki/NPH_insulin.

V. C. Medvei, "Chronological Tables," *History of Clinical Endocrinology* (Taylor & Francis, January 1, 1993), 488.

S.S. Londhe, "A Major Health Hazard: Metabolic Syndrome," *International Journal of Pharmacy and Pharmaceutical Sciences* (2011), ISSN-0975-1491, Vol. 3, Issue 3: 1-8.

Thebariatricsurgeryresource.com, *The History of Bariatric Surgery*, http://thebariatricsurgeryresource.com/articles/2012/03/06/history-bariatric-surgery.

Wikipedia.org, *Metformin*, http://en.wikipedia.org/wiki/Metformin.

"Science: Simulated ACTH," *Time*, December 12, 1960.

Citizendium.org, *Diabesity*, http://en.citizendium.org/wiki/Diabesity.

B.A. Ramlo-Halsted, S.V. Edelman, "The Natural History of Type 2 Diabetes: Practical Points to Consider in Developing Prevention and Treatment Strategies," *Clinical Diabetes* (2000), Vol. 18 No. 2: 80-84.

K. Tatemoto, "Neuropeptide Y: History and Overview", ed. M.C. Michel, *Neuropeptide Y and Related Peptides* (Springer, 2004): 2-12.

S. Zac-Varghese, T. Tan, S. R. Bloom, "Hormonal Interactions Between Gut and Brain," *Discovery Medicine* (Dec 26, 2010).

T. J. Kieffer, J. F. Habener, "The Glucagon-Like Peptides," *Endocrine Reviews* (December 1, 1999), doi: 10.1210/er.20.6.876, Vol. 20 No. 6: 876-913.

G.J. Cooper, A.C. Willis, A. Clark, et al., "Purification and characterization of a peptide from amyloid-rich pancreases of type 2 diabetic patients," Proceedings of the National Academy of Sciences of the United States of America (December 1987), PMCID: PMC299599: 8628–8632.

Wikipedia.org, *Leptin*, http://en.wikipedia.org/wiki/Leptin.

Medicalnews.net, *Metformin*, http://www.news-medical.net/health/Metformin-History.aspx.

Wikipedia.org, *Adiponectin*, http://en.wikipedia.org/wiki /Adiponectin.

Solomon Sobel, Director - Center For Drug Evaluation and Research, to Jennifer Stotka, Director, U.S. Regulatory Affairs – Eli Lilly and Company, September 11, 1998.

J.B. Hillman, J. Tong, M. Tschop, "Ghrelin Biology and Its Role in Weight-related Disorders," *Discovery Medicine* (June 17, 2011).

R. A. Pittner, A. A. Young, J. R. Paterniti, Jr., "Methods of treating obesity using PYY," U.S. Patent Application (December 14, 2001).

S.R. Bloom, et al., "Oxyntomodulin for preventing or treating excess weight," U.S. Patent Application (September 9, 2002).

M. Nauck, "Type 2 Diabetes: Principles and Practice, Second Edition," eds. B.J. Goldstein, D. Mueller-Wieland, *Type 2 Diabetes*, (CRC Press, November 14, 2007): 159.

T.E. Gottschalk Boeving, S. Klysner, "Immunization against autologous ghrelin," U.S. Patent Application (September 12, 2003).

"New GLP-1 analogs, mimetics in the pipeline for type 2 diabetes," *Endocrine Today*, May 2009.

M.C. Jones, "Therapies for Diabetes: Pramlintide and Exenatide," *American Family Physician* (June 15, 2007), 75(12): 1831-1836.

Bms.com, "U.S. FDA Grants Priority Review to Bristol-Myers Squibb and AstraZeneca's Metreleptin, an Investigational Agent for Treatment of Metabolic Disorders Associated with Rare Forms of Lipodystrophy," http://news.bms. com/press-release/us-fda-grants-priority-review-bristol-myers-squibb-and-astrazenecas-metreleptin-invest.

ACKNOWLEDGMENTS

I COULD NOT HAVE WRITTEN this book without the passion, trust, and commitment of all my patients. In the early years of my clinical practice at Seattle Performance Medicine, hundreds of patients faithfully tracked their food intake, hunger levels, exercise, and sleep. Together, we discovered that diets simply don't work long-term, and we searched for other, more successful, treatments. Some faced problems that were particularly difficult to diagnose, but they persisted as we worked to find and target their underlying metabolic glitches. Thanks to all of these patients, many others have benefited from what we learned along the path of discovery.

It takes great courage, curiosity, and determination to have faith in a new process. But my patients never stopped believing that, through science, we could diagnose and treat their underlying metabolic problems. And by understanding how their metabolism operated, they were finally freed from deprivation dieting forever.

It also takes great courage to share a personal story. I am grateful for my patients who were willing to speak out so that readers with similar issues might know that they are not alone and that help is possible. I am especially grateful for my past patient, Bea, who convinced me twenty years ago that the body is capable of healing itself. Bea suffered from obesity and she nearly lost her life several times due to complications stemming from treatment she had received in the past. She inspired me to believe in the body's healing capabilities and to never underestimate its power to survive—and even thrive—in spite of extraordinarily adverse circumstances.

Thank you, Dr. Hans Lisser and the other 20th-century pioneers in the field of metabolism and obesity, for challenging popular assumptions with science and inspiring me to continue my search for new, science-based solutions to what is today our country's Diabesity Epidemic. And thank you, present-day experts, my colleagues, and my mentors. I value the insight, support, and inspiration you generously provide.

My family has always encouraged me to follow my dreams and be a brave explorer, even if my pursuits lead to facts that challenge the status quo. Thanks to my parents, Ed and Jan, for their unconditional love and their assurance that everything is possible, for encouraging me in all my endeavors, and for urging me to always seek the truth and act upon it, regardless of popular opinion. And to my sister, Laurie: I'm truly grateful for your constant love and support.

Thank you to my talented team—Andrea Taylor, Beret Hamilton, Molly Hendrickson, and Jan Cooper—whose tenacity, creativity, and focus brought this book to life. I couldn't have accomplished so much without you.

I am indebted to Joyce Taylor for her insight and compassion toward those affected with weight issues, and for generously providing a platform through which we are able to share exciting science showing that weight problems are actually metabolism problems—not the result of failed diets or lack of willpower.

Finally, I would like to acknowledge author Hilary Beard for her critical role in getting this book off the ground.

ABOUT THE AUTHOR

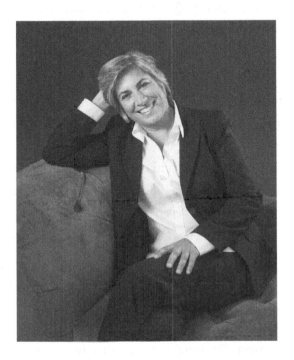

DR. EMILY COOPER, a Seattle-based physician with more than twenty years of experience, is board-certified in three specialties: Family Medicine, Sports Medicine, and Obesity Medicine. Dr. Cooper developed her clinical skills during medical school at London Hospital Medical College in England. There, she learned to combine an investigative approach with scientific analysis to obtain a comprehensive view of each of her patients.

In the late 1980s, while completing her residency at a community hospital in Pennsylvania, Dr. Cooper became interested in emerging research that associated several health conditions with increased body weight. She was excited to learn that metabolic imbalances such as metabolic syndrome and insulin resistance were most likely reversible and preventable. This opened up a new avenue for making a difference in preventing weight problems, diabetes, heart attacks, and strokes.

Dr. Cooper's interest in metabolism and obesity grew in the 1990s, when she realized that some of her patients were gaining weight even though they were trying to lose or maintain their weight. Looking back, she says she was naïve to think that all she needed to do to help her patients lose weight was to educate them about healthy eating and exercise. In spite of her efforts to perfect the "calories in, calories out" formula, individualizing it for each patient, Dr. Cooper found that regardless of how much weight a patient lost, it always came back.

Dr. Cooper's persistence over the past twenty years has led her to challenge antiquated assumptions and embrace a scientific perspective with the goal of more effectively treating weight problems. Today, most of her patients have experienced significant improvements in their health, metabolism, and weight as a result of applying a scientific approach instead of engaging in dieting and exercise weight-loss strategies.

In the course of her work with patients and their families in her clinical practice, Seattle Performance Medicine, Dr. Cooper has become convinced that the evidence in support of a science-based approach to obesity and metabolic malfunction needs a stronger voice to gain the attention of the healthcare community, the media, and the general public.

In an effort to provide a sounding board for the science of metabolism and its importance in reversing the country's Diabesity Epidemic, Dr. Cooper founded The Diabesity Research Foundation, a non-profit organization. Health experts predict that the Diabesity Epidemic—a public health crisis characterized by the combined epidemics of obesity and type 2 diabetes—will affect up to 60 percent of the U.S. adult population by 2020. The Foundation's mandate is to increase public awareness of the science behind diabesity through research and education.

In Dr. Cooper's view, it is only by basing prevention and treatment on the underlying causes of obesity that we can achieve meaningful overall health. Dr. Cooper hopes that with a greater public awareness of the science of metabolism and obesity, we will move away from antiquated assumptions and ineffective, potentially harmful treatments and redirect our efforts towards the findings of pure science.

CPSIA information can be obtained at www.ICGtesting.com
Printed in the USA
LVOW03s1933080814

398205LV00012B/89/P